Food Policy and Practice in Early Childhood Education and Care

This book is about food and feeding in early childhood education and care, offering an exploration of the intersection of children's food, education, family intervention, and public health policies.

The notion of 'good' food for children is often communicated as a matter of common sense by policymakers and public health authorities; yet the social, material, and practical aspects of feeding children are far from straightforward. Drawing on a detailed ethnographic study conducted in a London nursery and children's centre, this book provides a close examination of the practices of childcare practitioners, children, and parents, asking how the universalism of policy and bureaucracy fits with the particularism of feeding and eating in the early years. Looking at the unintended consequences that emerged in the field, such as contradictory public health messaging and arbitrary policy interventions, the book reveals the harmful assumptions about disadvantaged groups that are perpetuated in policy discourse, and challenges the constructs of individual choice and responsibility as main determinants of health. Children's food practices at the nursery are examined to explore the notion that, whilst for adults it is what children eat that often matters most, to children it is how they eat that is more important. This book contributes to a growing body of literature evidencing how children's food is a contested domain, in which power relations are continuously negotiated. This raises questions not only on how children can be included in policy beyond a tokenistic involvement but also on what children's well-being might mean beyond the biomedical sphere.

The book will particularly appeal to students and scholars in food and health, food policy, childhood studies, and medical anthropology. Policymakers and non-governmental bodies working in the domains of children's food and early years policies will also find this book of interest.

Francesca Vaghi is an anthropologist and childhood studies scholar. She holds a PhD in anthropology and sociology from SOAS, University of London, and is currently a Research Associate at the School of Social Work & Social Policy at the University of Strathclyde, Scotland. Francesca's work seeks to advance critical approaches in public health, specifically looking at how dominant policy discourses (re)create and seek to address 'problems' that have implications for working class and ethnic minority families, particularly in matters related to food insecurity, childhood poverty, and childcare policy.

Routledge Food Studies

Food Education and Gastronomic Tradition in Japan and France
Ethical and Sociological Theories
Haruka Ueda

Finding Meaning in Wine
A US Blend
Michael Sinowitz

Food Policy and Practice in Early Childhood Education and Care
Children, Practitioners, and Parents in an English Nursery
Francesca Vaghi

For more information about this series, please visit: www.routledge.com/
Routledge-Food-Studies/book-series/RFOODS

Food Policy and Practice in Early Childhood Education and Care

Children, Practitioners, and Parents in an English Nursery

Francesca Vaghi

Routledge
Taylor & Francis Group
LONDON AND NEW YORK

earthscan
from Routledge

First published 2024
by Routledge
4 Park Square, Milton Park, Abingdon, Oxon OX14 4RN

and by Routledge
605 Third Avenue, New York, NY 10158

Routledge is an imprint of the Taylor & Francis Group, an informa business

© 2024 Francesca Vaghi

The right of Francesca Vaghi to be identified as author of this work has been asserted in accordance with sections 77 and 78 of the Copyright, Designs and Patents Act 1988.

Trademark notice: Product or corporate names may be trademarks or registered trademarks, and are used only for identification and explanation without intent to infringe.

British Library Cataloguing-in-Publication Data
A catalogue record for this book is available from the British Library

ISBN: 978-1-032-28609-9 (hbk)
ISBN: 978-1-032-28610-5 (pbk)
ISBN: 978-1-003-29764-2 (ebk)

DOI: 10.4324/9781003297642

Typeset in Times New Roman
by codeMantra

To my parents.

Contents

Figures

Acknowledgements

My deep gratitude goes, first and foremost, to the children, early years practitioners, and parents who so generously welcomed me into their community between 2016 and 2017. Thank you for sharing your time, struggles, thoughts, and food (!) with me. It is my hope that what I have written here will do justice to your experiences and points of view.

I am infinitely grateful to my PhD supervisors, Professor Rebecca O'Connell and Dr Elizabeth Hull, for your selflessness, encouragement, and kindness – you are exceptional academics and people, who helped me grow into a stronger scholar. I feel very fortunate to have worked alongside you, and dearly miss our regular conversations. I would also like to thank Professor Harry West, for the vital input at the start of my doctoral studies. Thanks to my PhD examiners, Professor Samantha Punch and Professor Vicky Johnson, for helping me refine my arguments and writing; looking back on your feedback and advice was indispensable as I turned my thesis into this book. Thanks to Hannah Ferguson and Katie Stokes at Routledge, for your editorial input. I would also like to give thanks to the funding body that sponsored my doctoral research, the Bloomsbury Colleges, for the generous PhD studentship awarded to me.

Thanks to my parents, Monica Mezzalama and Riccardo Vaghi, for your infinite support and belief in me. To my brother, Fede Vaghi, thanks for sharing those London years with me and for being my rock during my doctoral studies.

To my chosen family, Craig Beyerinck and Pia Noel, I cannot express the extent of my gratitude for your friendship, love, and care, and for your input on the many drafts this piece of work has been through. I am deeply thankful to Furtuna Sheremeti, for your unending encouragement, friendship, and for always being an inspiration to me and others. A special thank you also goes to Imran Jamal, for your invaluable advice on all things anthropology and life related, and your feedback on numerous chapters of this book.

I am grateful to friends and colleagues at SOAS and the Thomas Coram Research Unit, who supported me and provided feedback on my work between 2015 and 2019, especially Celia Plender, Zofia Boni, Katharina Graf, Caro Gutierrez, Pavel Rubio, and Merve Uzunalioglu. I would like to particularly thank Alina Apostu, without whom I would not have been able to arrive (somewhat!) painlessly at the overarching argument in this book.

To the many, many other friends, family, and colleagues who have supported and encouraged me throughout the years it has taken for this book to be written: thank you. I am especially grateful to Stina Wassén, Thomas Feige, Siiri Sjöstrand-Kingdom, Léa Duchemin, Carl Truedsson, Thuy Phan, Iben Merrild, Sara O'Brien, Katherine Long, Rachel McNally, Eric Latorre, Thaddeus Castillo, Lara Wehbe, Eefje Vaghi, Lella Vaghi, and Giorgio Rigamonti. I would like to particularly thank Kathryn Nash, for coming to my rescue so many times as I completed this project.

A final, enormous thank you goes to my partner, Julia Hvitlock, for your patience and love, and for helping me untangle my thoughts, about this book and so much more.

Acronyms and abbreviations

EBSB	Eat Better Start Better Framework
ECEC	Early Childhood Education and Care
EYFS	Statutory Framework for the Early Years Foundation Stage
HENRY	The HENRY (Health, Exercise, Nutrition for the Really Young) Approach
MEW	Mixed Economy of Welfare
NHS	National Health Service
WPR	What's the Problem Represented to Be? Approach

Introduction

It is a spring morning in London. A group of five mothers, their children, two early years practitioners, and I, are sitting around a table at Ladybird Nursery and Children's Centre.[1] We are participating in one of six 'healthy cooking'[2] sessions that a local food advocacy charity is delivering to families registered with the children's centre. Sat on our child-sized chairs and equipped with plastic knives and chopping boards, we cut the ingredients needed to cook that day's recipe, assisted by the chef employed by the charity and a volunteer assistant, who are running the session. As we animatedly go about our tasks, three-year-old Sam approaches his mother Aida and furtively begins poking at her handbag, which hangs near her hip. She initially tries to stop him from unzipping the bag, but her attempts to do so immediately upset him, so she concedes. While Sam dives his hand into his mother's handbag with precise intention, Aida explains to us, embarrassed, that he is looking for Tic Tac's,[3] a couple of which he eats with delight, before his mother takes them back from him and puts them away. The chef, who is also sitting with us, smiles at her: "We're not judging," she says reassuringly. The volunteer assistant adds, "It's ok, he ate some fruit before!"[4] These comments do not appear to console Aida, who seems mortified by what just happened. Some of the other mothers offer her supportive glances, but no one else says anything, and the session carries on.

It is not the first time that brief, but poignant, moments of tension such as this one happen during the cooking class. The chef's comment to Aida – "We're not judging" – is unintentionally ironic. In England, cooking courses like today's are offered in state-maintained early years settings precisely because some parents' feeding and eating practices have been judged as deficient by policymakers. In particular, the assumption that low-income families lack the knowledge and skills to properly feed their children prevails in official discourse, and indeed this is the group to whom such interventions are regularly promoted. These initiatives, which emerge at the intersection of public health, family intervention, and early childhood education and care (ECEC) policies, tend to obscure the numerous and interlinking constraints that parents face when feeding their children. For Aida, for example, knowledge and skills are not an issue: over the couple of weeks that we have spent together, she has told me a lot about the food she cooks at home for her family, and the time and labour that some of the dishes she makes require. The problem she has faced since moving to London from Eastern Europe, she told me, is being able

DOI: 10.4324/9781003297642-1

to afford to buy all the ingredients that she needs to cook for her three sons and husband, relying solely on her husband's salary.

Yet, circumstances such as Aida's are rarely taken into account in the initiatives and discussions that I encountered during my year of fieldwork. Aida knows that what children eat and are fed is under constant scrutiny, and that Sam's way of taking sweets from her handbag reveals that this is common practice between them. Her reaction during this episode might seem extreme, but in a context in which parents – especially mothers – are widely held responsible for their children's diets, her uneasiness is warranted.

Linked to these assumptions is also the preconception that adults influence children's diets in a unidirectional and authoritative way that goes unchallenged by children. Nonetheless, children – who otherwise have little control over most aspects that impact their daily lives – regularly contest adult attempts to regulate their diets, and develop their own preferences and attitudes towards food from an early age. An emphasis on food's 'healthiness' also obscures the social and caring role that food plays in child-adult relations. The volunteer's comment to Aida reveals that food and eating are inherently moral – it is ok if Sam eats some Tic Tac's, because he had some fruit earlier. The 'good' cancels out the 'bad.'

In framing food as 'healthy' or 'unhealthy,' attention is paid to *what* children are fed, but less so to *how* they are fed and *how* they eat. This has implications within households, but also institutions. Some of the staff at Ladybird also attend the cooking course that Aida and I are taking part in, and regularly go to training sessions promoted by the local council to improve early years practitioners' knowledge and skills. This, by and large, reflects the emphasis that British policymakers have given to early intervention in the last decades, as well as the aims put forward in the voluntary food guidelines that most early years settings in England abide by. Simultaneously, providing 'good' food to children at nursery links to the assumption that early years services compensate for perceived shortcomings within the home environment.

This book is about children's food policy and practice in early childhood education and care (ECEC). By exploring how early years settings in England have emerged as sites where public health, education, and family intervention policies intertwine, I argue that the universalism of policy and bureaucracy sits uncomfortably alongside the particularism that feeding children (at home and within institutions) entails.

Whilst this overarching argument might seem succinct, the questions I asked to arrive at it explored the complexity that lies at the heart of all matters related to feeding children in the early years. When examining policy, I wanted to know, what 'problems' related to children's eating are considered most pressing by official actors? What factors are perceived to be making these 'problems' persist? And what is the historical context that has contributed to certain assumptions to prevail in official and mainstream narratives about children's food? These questions, in turn, also revealed what is left out of these discourses, and the impact that these policy framings of the 'problems' have on the lives of children, parents, carers, and those working in the early years.

To understand this last aspect of my research – how policy impacts on people's everyday lives – I first explored how official and mainstream discourses were engaged with and put into practice by practitioners at Ladybird, as well as other official actors who operated in the setting (like local government officials, medical professionals, and those working for the charity sector). I asked, what are the aims of feeding children (in an early years setting and at home), and what does feeding children involve? Adults who cared for children often found themselves having to balance a number of practical and logistical aims (and bureaucratic aims, if within the early years setting) with their own particular set of values, values which at times did not align with those of other adults'. The question of whose responsibility it is to feed children (particularly to feed them 'healthy' food) was also salient in these conversations, echoing policy and mainstream rhetoric about children's food.

And, when considering all these questions, I also wanted to know what are children's viewpoints and experiences of mealtimes? It is generally assumed that adults influence children's eating in a unidirectional and authoritative way, however, when exploring children's everyday practices, it becomes apparent that this is not the case. What strategies do children use to contest and overturn adult rules and norms about food and eating? What practices do children bring from their home environment to the school, and vice versa? What do children value about food and mealtimes? And how can these insights help inform policy and practice?

Challenging universalism: anthropological approaches in policy analysis

Policy and bureaucracy regulate daily activities in early years settings, such as feeding and eating, but also the future 'outcomes' that children and parents should aspire to. Understanding the rationales that inform policies and policymakers' decisions is crucial (Wedel et al. 2005, 34). This sheds light on a contradiction still inherent in much of contemporary policymaking: the assumption that policies function as a kind of 'assembly line,' with a direct cause-and-effect, ignoring the much deeper complexity of the social fabric they aim to intervene on (ibid., 38). Equally important is to ask how 'problems' are represented in official discourse (Bacchi and Goodwin 2016). An ethnographic exploration of policy can thus help us challenge its presumed universalism, by bringing the particularism of daily life to the fore.

Questioning the assumption of policy as a rational mechanism also reveals that there is incongruity between understandings of policy on an abstract versus a practical level: what happens on the ground is rarely unidirectional. Writing about international development projects, Mosse asks: "What if, instead of policy producing practice, practices produce policy, in the sense that actors in development devote their energies to maintaining coherent representations regardless of events?" (2005, 2). In the context of my research, as I will show, there were several mechanisms in place to ensure that official actors were being given evidence that policies and interventions were being implemented at Ladybird – even if the day-to-day practices and outcomes were not as neat, linear, or measurable as expected.

The implementation of certain initiatives within Ladybird – both with children and parents – revealed how a mismatch between intention and outcomes can take place. On one hand, work by official actors is indeed frequently carried out with the best of intentions; on the other, assumptions about so-called 'target groups' (often bolstered by policy itself) can also clash with these motives, and the pressures generated by England's audit culture (Power 1999; Strathern 2000; Shore 2017) seem to perpetuate some of the failures that policies attempt to rectify. As Mosse argues, most official bodies "are bound to a managerial view of policy which makes them resolutely simplistic about (or ignorant of) the social and political life of their ideas" (2005, 20). Institutions and organisations need to maintain a veneer of coherence when promoting policy initiatives, to secure funds that will enable them to continue operating. Yet, these funds do not necessarily guarantee that interventions will be 'successful.' In this sense, the gap between policy and practices 'on the ground' become politically necessary (ibid., 7) – policies (often informed by inaccurate assumptions) will continue to be developed and deployed, because the 'problems' they seek to address will also continue to exist.

An ethnography of policy can help us investigate why certain inequalities persist, despite repeated and renewed interventions to tackle them by local and national governments. In the context of Uttar Pradesh, Gupta contends that structural violence in India is not a result of official actors' indifference or ill-intentions, but of the haphazard way in which bureaucracy operates by nature (2012, 6). In Gupta's work, the fundamental question is why it is state bureaucracy that creates arbitrariness in the first place (ibid., 24). He contends that researching everyday bureaucratic practices is essential to understand why structural violence persists, is upheld by bureaucracy itself, "and why, paradoxically, [violence] is often found in practices of welfare" (ibid., 31). In my research, I observed how national and local policies also worked in this contradictory way. At the time I began my fieldwork in the summer of 2016, it seemed urgent to explore these issues; decades of austerity politics (Ridge 2013; Loopstra et al. 2015; McKenzie 2015; Stuckler et al. 2017; Edminston 2018) weighed heavily on the early years sector in England, impacting food provision within settings. Britain had also just fallen into an unknown and unstable territory following the results of the Brexit referendum. The exit of Britain from the European Union was predicted to have severe impact on food supply, affordability, and quality (Lang et al. 2018; Lang 2019), and indeed this prediction could not have been more correct (e.g. Millstone, Lang, and Marsden 2019; Strong and Wells 2020; Hlaimi 2021). Yet, policy paradigms seem to not have evolved parallel to these immense structural and geopolitical shocks.

Governmentality: food, families, and children

U.K. policymaking has been largely shaped by advanced liberalism, a context where the state's main role has increasingly become to produce rational, independent citizens who can make the 'right' choices, rather than being a main provider of welfare services (Moss and Petrie 2000, 50). It is important to clarify that whilst many of the authors I will quote refer to this political ideology as 'neoliberalism,' I have chosen the term 'advanced liberalism' to be more precise about the conditions that shaped the context in which my research is situated. The term neoliberalism (widely) connotes ideals of (free-)marketisation, privatisation, and state de-regulation most commonly associated with conservatism (Peck and Theodore 2012). Nonetheless, as I will discuss, such features in Britain's sociopolitical system did not only emerge during Conservative (right-wing) administrations, but also under left-wing governments, particularly during the New Labour years (1997–2010). I thus align myself with Rose and Lentzos, who argue that:

> The attack on the rationalities of welfare came not just from the right but from all sides of the political spectrum: from the left, who argued that the welfare state, despite its apparent egalitarianism, actually enshrined inequality and generated a powerful and unregulated welfare bureaucracy whose primary function was social control; and from classical liberals with their concern for individual rights, who argued that the powers of professional expertise within the welfare apparatus violated rights and substituted professional discretion for due process. Almost all seemed to agree that state-organized welfare services, as they actually existed, destroyed informal practices of solidarity and social support, enshrined professional power, and produced clientism rather than socially responsible citizens.
>
> (2017, 32)

This rationale has shaped much of the rhetoric inherent in policies that impact on children's lives – be it related to food, ECEC, or family intervention. Advanced liberalism has also largely shaped what Powell (2014) has described as Britain's Mixed Economy of Welfare (MEW), or Welfare Pluralism, a system which comprises state, market, and voluntary (or informal) elements in the provision of welfare services (2014, 2). For the domain of ECEC, for example, several scholars have already discussed the effect of the increasing marketization and fragmentation of childcare services in Britain (e.g. Randall 2004; Penn 2011), which promoted a focus on competition between providers and quality evaluations, largely consequent to the consolidation of an 'audit culture' (Power 1999; Strathern 2000; Shore 2017) in Britain since the 1990s.

The advanced liberal state's success in shaping citizens who are autonomous, responsible, and rational relies in great part on the process that Foucault described as 'governmentality.' In 'Technologies of the Self' (1988), Foucault identifies four "specific techniques that human beings use to understand themselves" (1988, 18): technologies of production, technologies of sign systems, technologies of power, and technologies of the self. Technologies of power, he contends, "determine the conduct of individuals and submit them to certain ends or domination" (ibid.), whilst technologies of the self "permit individuals to effect by their own means or with the help of others a certain number of operations on their own bodies and souls, thoughts, conduct, and way of being" (ibid.). The interaction between these two technologies in particular, he puts forward, is what constitutes governmentality (ibid., 19).

These techniques are fundamental for states to govern populations under advanced liberalism. By regulating most aspects of daily life through policies and mechanisms enacted within different governmental and non-governmental organizations, and by relying on individuals' self-surveillance, the state can govern populations "at a distance" (ibid., 57). This is echoed by Shore and Wright (1997), who argue that policies, central to "modern power" (ibid., 7), are 'political technologies' that allow for the act of government to be conducted in this 'distant' way. Under advanced liberalism, the notion of 'expertise' is fundamental to enact governmentality (Rose 1996, 50; Shore and Wright 1997, 8–9). Within this paradigm, authority and 'expertise' are deeply tied together, and even more so in the domains of food policy and public health.

Thinking of children's food, ECEC, and family intervention policies using a Foucauldian lens helps reveal how different authoritative voices within these policy domains assert themselves, and what claims to 'expertise' each of them makes. Food, childhood, and family are all spheres that particularly lend themselves to being regulated via the techniques of government described by Foucault. For the case of food, Coveney contends that "The combination of science and moral conduct – which in many ways forms the basis of governmentality – are never so apparent as in nutrition" (2000, 23). Similarly, building on Foucault's work about governmentality and biopower (1978),[5] Lupton argues that, "Public health and health promotion…may be viewed as contributing to the moral regulation of society, focusing as they do on upon ethical and moral practices of the self," with institutions working to shape citizens bound by limited and particular "moral judgements" (1995, 4–5). She further comments that,

> governmentality sees power relations as diffuse, as emerging not necessarily from the state but from all areas of social life [locating] regulatory activities at all levels of social institutions, from the family, the mass media and the school to national bureaucratic agencies.
>
> (ibid., 9)

As I will show in Chapter 1, on the macro-scale "regulatory activities" emerge in the wording of children's food policy, emphasising the relation between choice and health as well as the importance of successful early intervention for future outcomes. These, in turn, link to broader discourses in English policy about acceptable models of family life as well as personhood, which focus on individual choice. On the micro-scale, the "diffuse" quality of governmentality is apparent when hearing people's accounts of scrutinising their own as well as others' practices, something that I will particularly focus on in Chapters 5 and 6 of this book.

Foucault's and Lupton's framing of governmentality as "diffuse" (Foucault 1991; Lupton 1995) thus helps us to bridge the gap between the macro- and micro-scales. Following Foucault's historical and philosophical contextualisation of technologies of the self as "types of self-examination" (1988, 46), it is important to explore not only how governmentality is enacted from the top-down, but also how it is enacted between individuals, and by individuals on themselves. As I will explore in this book, and as shown in the opening vignette of this Introduction, this was particularly the case for mothers, who often expressed feeling under pressure to feed their children the 'right' way. This anxiety seemed rooted both in a self-consciousness about one's *own* practices, but also in the awareness they had for *each other's* practices, and the moral judgements attached to these observations of oneself and others. The self-surveillance that governmentality entails is intrinsic to the notion that autonomous, rational, and responsible individuals can make 'good choices' about the food they eat (and feed to their children). These ideas of choice and responsibility manifested constantly during the year I carried out fieldwork. Not only were adults preoccupied with teaching children about 'healthy eating' so that they could learn to make these 'good choices' in the future, adults' behaviour and practices were subjected to this level of scrutiny.

Alongside the interaction between health and food policy, it is also crucial to think about how family intervention policy is conceived of in advanced liberalism: Foucault noted the centrality of the family as an "instrument for the government of the population" (1991, 100). Family life is an important sphere for policy intervention in the U.K., and policy assumptions about which families need to be intervened upon, and which do not, need to be closely examined (e.g. Macvarish in Lee et al. 2014). An example is New Labour government's Sure Start programme launched in 1998, which saw the inauguration of children's centres that offered educational initiatives (and other kinds of community support) to families with children under primary school age. Predominantly, Sure Start services were offered to 'target groups' comprised of unemployed, low-income, and lone parents (Clarke 2006, 705), with the long-term aim of tackling poverty and 'social exclusion' (ibid., 700).

In this book, I have thus chosen to explore family life, education, and public health as three of the key domains through which governmentality is enacted. Within each of these spheres, children become 'subjects' of different interventions that aim to produce a particular kind of citizen (Moss and Petrie 2000, 65). This has direct consequences on the rationales that guide ECEC policy and provision, in which children are perceived as "economic units" (Gibson, McArdle, and Hatcher 2015), valuable for their expected future contributions. Yet, whilst studying children and childhood within advanced liberalism reveals how the entrenchment of this market-oriented ideology persists and prevails, it also provides an avenue to explore how resistance to it occurs, and invites us to imagine possible alternatives to the status quo (Moss 2015).

ECEC policy rationales

In Britain, significant developments in childcare policy took place during the post-World War II era, and the legacy of these changes continues to have significant impact on current assumptions that shape this policy domain. In the seminal book, *The Politics of Childcare in Britain* (2000), Randall argues that much of what has (or has not) determined childcare legislation in the U.K. is related to "a powerful 'ideology of motherhood,' or maternalism, which still exercises considerable informal influence" (ibid., 13). In the immediate years after World War II, nursery education and childcare, which had fulfilled the specific purpose of allowing mothers to take up work during the conflict, were no longer in the policymaking spotlight; an opportunity to establish universal and free early years services was lost (ibid., 52–53).

Randall further argues that, relative to other welfare states in Europe, the U.K. has given little priority to the establishment of reliable childcare services. She attributes this to the government's "(partial) incorporation of a liberal philosophy…and strong male breadwinner assumptions" (2002, 219) in the post-War years. Randall suggests that, thereafter, ECEC policy has tended to be changeable and inconsistent because the main beneficiaries of these policies (particularly at their inception) were women and children, a group without "political organization or leverage" (ibid., 224).[6] Randall further shows that ECEC has always been a particularly fragmented policy domain, with a tension between childcare and early education (2002, 220–25), but also historically between education and public health (2000, 54), which further blurs the aims and outcomes sought by official actors when developing legislation.

The ruptured and muddy nature of the ECEC policy context has created a fruitful environment for the proliferation of a more market-oriented model of childcare provision in Britain. This has created a wide array of childcare options, a 'mixed economy of childcare' (Moss and Petrie 2000; Lewis 2013). Randall's assessment of the state as a 'regulator' or 'coordinator' of childcare services, rather than a 'direct provider' (2002, 220), is thus still the model currently in place in the U.K. at large. In England, ECEC is offered by a number of providers: private (for-profit) day nurseries, voluntary (not-for-profit) day nurseries, state-maintained (or state-funded) nursery schools, nursery and reception classes attached to primary schools, playgroups, and childminders[7] (Department for Education 2016, 5). At the time during which I carried out my fieldwork, there were 54 nursery schools in the borough, only two of which were state-maintained – Ladybird was one of these two.

An increasingly privatised, market-driven ECEC sector is a result of (and further results in) the fragmentation of this policy domain, and the myriad rationales and interests that childcare policy is linked to. And, influenced by the advanced liberal paradigm that has prevailed in British politics since the 1980s, two of the key rationales underpinning the development of childcare policy is that provision of early years services should help boost parental employment and improve children's school readiness (Moss and Petrie 2000; Randall 2000; Penn 2007, 2011; Platt 2007; Moss 2012).

The link between childcare provision and parental employment has been a central driver of ECEC policy advancements since the post-War era (Randall 2002). As indicated under the 'Aims' section of the Department of Education's Childcare Bill, "Additional free childcare will help families by reducing the cost of childcare and will support parents into work or to work more hours" (Department of Education 2015, 4). Increasing parents' – and specifically mothers' – participation in the economy is framed as one of the components of a larger 'government productivity plan' which aims to reduce "unfair or distorting barriers to work, including women whose high levels of skills are too often underused" (ibid.). Early years practitioners and scholars alike have questioned the goal of boosting parental employment through childcare provision without providing adequate funding to ECEC settings.

For example, a recent development to ECEC policy related to increasing parental employment and reducing poverty has been the 30-hours free childcare allowance[8] for three- and four-year-olds with working parents,[9] which came into effect in England in September 2017 (Goodwill 2017). Early trials of the scheme, however, showed that the childcare sector was not ready to implement the scheme, due to insufficient numbers of staff (Pre-school Learning Alliance 2017, 3). Families also began to be charged for goods and services that were previously being provided to children for free (ibid.), including food. A further unintended consequence of the 30-hours allowance was that children of unemployed parents (and thus who are less likely to be able to afford any form of childcare) were not able to access the same levels of childcare hours as before the policy was rolled out.

Making changes to policy without adequately addressing structural issues reflects a broader and crucial contradiction in childcare policy (in the U.K. and across the world): while the early years are framed as a crucial time for children's development and well-being, ECEC also tends to be a domain that is underinvested in (Michel 2002, 334). Moss and Petrie have argued that efforts to reduce poverty by boosting parental employment without addressing issues of structural social inequality tend to be futile (2000, 82). Further, this leads to children's well-being being viewed predominantly in relation to their parents' employment status, rather than as also linked to the quality of their daily experiences in childcare (ibid.).

Preparing children for primary education has also increasingly become a central aim of ECEC policy. Improved school readiness is mentioned as one of the intended outcomes of the Childcare Bill[10] (Department for Education 2015, 27, 132, 145) and is emphasised throughout the 'Statutory framework for the early years foundation stage' (EYFS) (Department for Education 2017). In the Childcare Bill, the benefit of children being enrolled in some form of early years service is discussed in terms of 'positive future outcomes' (2015, 19).

The future-oriented language of ECEC policy needs to be questioned. Qvortrup, for example, has argued that this reinforces a view of children as 'becomings' rather than 'beings,' valuable mainly for their potential as future adults (2005, 5). Mayall contends that emphasis on future outcomes and preparedness for further education is a result of a "continued dominance in the U.K. of positivist development psychology" that frames children as "socialisation projects" (2006, 13). Others suggest that, under advanced liberalism, ECEC just becomes another mechanism through which children can be shaped into future (productive) citizens (Moss and Petrie 2000, 62).

Emphasis on future outcomes – whether educational or behavioural – is not only intrinsic to much of ECEC policy discourse, but also to the rhetoric around public health and children's food. Drawing attention away from children's present experiences in childcare, by emphasising parental employment and school readiness, can lead to contradictions and unintended consequences in policy interventions, as well as a conflation of policy objectives. This fraught policy landscape has direct impact on people's practices on the ground, particularly when policy and bureaucratic frameworks do not align with people's ethics of care.

The ethics of care: universalism vs. particularism

This book draws predominantly from the works of feminist scholars to explore the concept of caring through food, particularly Tronto (1993, 2013) and Abel and Nelson (1990). Tronto's definition of care emphasises its practical dimension, and the link between thought and action that caring practices require (1993, 108). Tronto challenges the notion that carework is straightforward, or that it requires little skill or training. She contends that this is one of the contradictions inherent in how care is thought of, perceived as simultaneously essential and marginal to our daily lives (ibid., 111). A parallel can be drawn here with food. Aside to being necessary for our survival, eating is central to our sense of identity, well-being, and social belonging (Lupton 1996, 36), yet it is also often a taken for granted sphere in the everyday. In ECEC policy discourse, what children eat is considered fundamental, but nutritional guidelines can be vague, or resources to fulfil them insufficient. Similarly, in official discourse it is assumed that parents always can and want to dedicate significant time and money to feeding their children (O'Connell and Brannen 2016, 82), when in fact this might also not be possible for a plethora of reasons (e.g. employment commitments, fuel poverty, lack of access to adequate food suppliers, etc.).

Like Tronto, Abel and Nelson show the seemingly opposing elements that are reconciled by, and through, caring practices. They argue that "good care" needs to encourage the autonomy of those being cared for, whilst also recognising their position of dependence (1990, 5). "Good care" bridges the gap between public and private, and "challenges the division between reason and emotion" (ibid.). They further argue that "bureaucratic norms of impersonality and emotional distance are reinforced" through professionalism (ibid., 13),[11] so that caregivers' personal experiences and knowledge(s) are devalued in the caregiving encounter. Importantly, Abel and Nelson contend that there is a "conflict between the universalism of bureaucracies and the particularism of caregiving" (ibid., 12), arguing that "Caregiving fits uneasily into bureaucracies" because institutions "operate on the basis of a set of general rules, but the essence of caregiving is attentiveness to the individual" (ibid.). At Ladybird, staff's personal ethics of care often stood in contrast with the guidelines, regulations, and goals they were asked to follow. This tension – between the universalism of policy and bureaucracy and the particularism of feeding and eating – has been at the centre of my ethnographic findings, and each chapter will unpack this theme from a different perspective.

Bakhtin and the dialogic

Alongside (and complementary to) the ethics of care, Mikhail Bakhtin's work on the dialogic (1981, 1986) was particularly useful to explore micro-level exchanges between children, and between children and adults. Dialogism, as defined by Bakhtin, refers to,

> [the] constant interaction between meanings, all of which have the potential of conditioning others. Which will affect the other, how it will do so and in what degree is what is actually settled at the moment of utterance. This

dialogic imperative, mandated by the pre-existence of the language world...
insures that there can be no actual monologue.

(1981, 426)

Just as care is considered a relational concept in this book, so is Bakhtin's
dialogism. Bakhtin contends that everyday dialogue is inherently *responsive* (ibid.,
281). Any given 'utterance' or 'speech act' is conditioned by previous ones, and by
the responses the speaker expects from their interlocutor(s) (ibid., 282). Like the
ethics of care, dialogism encourages us to think of discourse and practice as always
co-produced (Mayerfeld Bell 1998, 59). I thus suggest that dialogism advances
our understanding of the continuity and interconnectedness that I explore between
policy, adults', and children's practices. Much of the literature exploring food and
governmentality in schools assesses top-down dynamics from the perspective of
children (e.g. Vander Schee 2009; Evans et al. 2011). Other authors have looked at
parents' (often subordinate) position when targeted for school food interventions,
sometimes alongside their children (e.g. Maher, Fraser, and Wright 2010; Maher,
Fraser, and Lindsay 2010; Pike and Leahy 2012). The concept of 'biopedagogy'
has also been used to show how surveillance of students takes place through food
education projects, both within schools but also at the interface of the school and
home environments (e.g. Leahy 2014; Petherick 2015; Leahy and Wright 2016).
Yet, in these framings of the issue, encounters with policy narratives are often
portrayed as unidirectional, and children's (and parents') positions vis-a-vis these
discourses needs further assessment.

Using a Bakhtinian lens can help problematise the assumed linearity between
policy and 'outcomes' on the ground, but also offers a counter-point to the assumption that adults influence children's practices in a unidirectional way. As I will
show, children's speech acts and practices at Ladybird – co-created in a circular
(dialogic) manner within peer groups – offered a way to contest adult attempts to
control their behaviour during mealtimes. Similarly, the norms about food and eating that children valued in school were often brought into the home environment:
parents' practices were also shaped by children, not just by official discourses.
Bakhtin's work thus provided a language for navigating the very different scales at
which the discourses and practices that I explore in my work unfolded: it was necessary to bring the analysis down to the level of minute communicative action and
linguistic exchanges, what Bakhtin called the 'moment of utterance' (1981, 426). A
focus at this level justifies the use of ethnographic methods as well.

Examining dialogic processes sheds light on the messiness and unpredictability
of everyday life, and of caring through food. Mol emphasises that care practices
are anything but linear, and dealing with the unexpected consequences of caring
encounters is an inherent component of what constitutes 'good' care (2008, 12).
Importantly, Mol argues that studying the 'logic of care' is a useful way to explore
how individualist norms promoted in advanced liberal paradigms can be challenged:

Care is a process: it does not have clear boundaries. It is open-ended [...]
it is a matter of time [...] Care is not a transaction in which something is

exchanged (a product against a price): but an interaction in which the action goes back and forth (in an ongoing process).

(ibid., 18)

By drawing on Bakhtin's work, I aim to explore this 'back and forth action' between the realms that I examine in this book – policy, children's, and adults' practices – and the consequences of not acknowledging (or valuing) this continuity of caring relations in official discourse.

Lessons from childhood studies

In *Making Sense of Everyday Life* (2009) Scott calls for the development of research approaches that uncover the relevance of daily routines to make sense of the mundane (2009, 4). Within this ongoing pursuit of the social sciences, however, children have not always been adequately considered or represented. Anthropologists have included children in their work as early as the 19th century (Montgomery 2009, 1), and famously in Margaret Mead's *Coming of Age in Samoa* (1928). Yet, the anthropology of childhood as a subfield was established in more recent decades, and not many scholars are working specifically on the early years (e.g. DeLoache and Gottlieb 2000; Gottlieb 2004).

This subfield in anthropology is indebted in large part to childhood studies, which challenged traditional conceptualisations of the child emerging from developmental psychology, with its premise that children 'internalise society' through the process of socialisation (Corsaro 2011, 9). Sociologists began to contest these notions in the late 1980s and 1990s, concretised by the 'paradigm shift' proposed by James and Prout (1997). These authors called for an increased awareness of children as agents, who are actively participating in the creation of the social worlds and relationships they engage in. This new model aimed to provide a theoretical and methodological means by which to gain access to, and develop, knowledge about children and childhood that was not derived from adult perspectives but by children themselves.

Anthropologists of childhood have shown that framing children as producers of meaningful knowledge about the everyday is an opportunity to refine the discipline as a whole (Toren 2007, 27), and particularly to challenge the vision of a universal progression from childhood to adulthood (Bluebond-Langner and Korbin 2007, 242), intimating that not only children, but adults too, are 'becomings' throughout the lifecourse (Uprichard 2008). As such, anthropologists of childhood have explored children's knowledge production and social participation in different societies across the world (e.g. Toren 2007, 2011, 2012; Lancy 2008; Cooper 2013), and their position within traditionally 'adult' domains, such as conflict (e.g. West 2000; Utas 2003), spirituality (e.g. Gottlieb 1998; Toren 2007), and, indeed, food and eating practices (e.g. de Matos Viegas 2003; Boni 2017, 2023). In particular, I aim to emphasise that children's general lack of visibility in these 'adult' realms is even more salient in policy matters, where children's voices are rarely represented meaningfully. Yet, rather than viewing policy, adults' practices, and children's practices as separate, I contend that an exploration of these as interlinked can reveal not only the shortcomings of policy, but also the similarities in both children's and adults' views and practices.

Corsaro's work (2011, 2005) has been instrumental in furthering our knowledge of how young children construct their self-identities and establish peer relations. He claims that children's agency is intersubjective in nature and, importantly, built and reproduced in social groups and through specific, meaningful actions (2011, 43). This process is epitomised by his notion of 'interpretive reproduction,' which, contrary to the traditional view that children's socialisation is "about adaptation and internalization" (ibid., 20), proposes that children "creatively appropriate or take knowledge from the adult world" (ibid., 42) to form a sense of self, and to build relations with peers, as well as with adults. This, according to Corsaro, is what makes the study of children and childhood particularly relevant and urgent (ibid., 43). Further, he emphasises the importance of recognising that children's agency needs to be situated and researched with full acknowledgement of their generational position (ibid., 31).

Analysing intergenerational relations and bringing generational perspectives together is central to the study of childhood. Alanen and Mayall, proposing that childhood should be viewed as "a relational concept" (2001, 1; see also Alanen 2011), contend that the age and power divides that inevitably affect generational groups' interactions necessitate particular attention. Qvortrup, who views childhood as a "structural form" (2011, 23), extends this position by emphasising that "social parameters" (such as class, gender, and ethnicity) have different implications on people's lives depending on their position in any given generational order (ibid., 27). We are thus invited to view children, like adults, as agents who are negotiating their position and influencing change through time in a given social and historical context, but who are often further constrained by their age status (see also Vanderbeck and Worth 2015; Mannion 2018; Punch and Vanderbeck 2018). At the same time, whilst recognising that children's agency can be limited by their status in the generational order, studying the transmission of knowledge and practices between generations can also help us question the assumed unidirectionality (from older to younger people) in these exchanges (Vanderbeck and Worth 2015, 6).

Understanding children's social participation and meaning making through food and eating can thus not only challenge the universalism of policy and bureaucracy but also contribute to the way childhood is viewed in official and mainstream discourse. Qvortrup argues that the notion of the 'modern child' is one marked by invisibility,[12] consequent to "a strong tendency to believe that the individual child and children as a group do not relate to adults in general, but only to their parents, teachers and supervisors" (Qvortrup 2005, 4). Qvortrup's analysis highlights a crucial paradox. He argues that although children's needs and agency have been given increasing recognition since the paradigm shift in childhood studies (James and Prout 1997), children and young people are often still not perceived as relevant contributors to their social worlds.

This tension becomes particularly salient when studying generational relations within institutional settings, and has been well documented by scholars working on children's food practices in these contexts. Jo Pike's work, for example, has examined the negotiation of power relations between adults and children during school meals using a Foucauldian lens (Pike 2008; Pike 2010; Pike and Leahy 2012), showing how discipline and resistance can simultaneously reaffirm but also contest generational hierarchies. By a similar token, ethnographies focusing on children's food practices in residential care illustrate that 'family-like' interactions within these settings (like mealtimes) muddy the meaning of care and caring (see for example Dorrer et al. 2010; Punch, McIntosh, and Emond 2012; Punch and McIntosh 2014; McIntosh et al. 2015; Cox et al. 2017). These works show how relations of care (through food) can be constrained by institutional and bureaucratic norms, and challenge how we might think about children's well-being and identities in relation to food and mealtimes.

An ethnographic case study of inner-London

In the last two decades, London's socio-economic contrasts (e.g. Butler, Hamnett, and Ramsden 2008; Hall 2008), and cultural and ethnic diversity have received particular attention in social science, especially the topics of multiculturalism, migration, and 'super-diversity' (e.g. Vertovec 2007; Alexander 2011; Berg and Sigona 2013; Wessendorf 2014; Back and Sinha 2018). The themes explored in these bodies of work reflect many of the demographic trends that have also happened in the borough where I chose to conduct ethnographic fieldwork between 2016 and 2017. The ethnically and culturally diverse population of my fieldsite, and its changing socio-economic fabric (visible also in the ongoing process of gentrification that the area has been experiencing in the last decades) largely mirror shifts that are taking place across the city. Of the 139 children (aged three- to four-years-old) enrolled at Ladybird Nursery during the 2016–2017 academic year, there were 20 different stated ethnicities and nationalities.[13]

The topic of minority groups' food practices has increasingly gained attention in England (e.g. Sarwar 2002; Chowbey and Harrop 2016) as well as in other countries (e.g. Akresh 2007; Halkier and Jensen 2011; Nielsen, Krasnik, and Holm 2013). Identifying a setting where cultural and ethnic diversity were prevalent was important to shed light on the tensions that emerge when different notions of 'good' food interact with one another. Policy and mainstream norms about food and eating often did not match the practices that children brought with them into the nursery setting, as I will show. Importantly, exploring daily life in a diverse context such as Ladybird's shows that those that hold authoritative voices in English policy communities often do not fully represent or engage with the various perspectives and knowledge(s) of the people to whom policies are promoted.

I was also particularly interested in exploring the impact of socio-economic inequality on children's access to adequate food, both within an institutional setting and in households. The borough in which Ladybird is found is among the most highly deprived local authorities in England (Department for Communities and Local Government 2015, 2019). Parallel to this, however, the area is also experiencing rapid economic growth, gentrification, and an influx of high-earning professionals moving into the area. This creates stark contrasts, reflected visibly in the urban landscape: social housing next to new private developments, or shut-down local businesses facing new 'trendier' shops and eateries catering to the wealthier members of the borough's population. Caraher and Dowler have argued that, in London, the starkest sign of inequality is food: "Those who are poor often have problems accessing food shops, affording a healthy diet and being part of mainstream food culture and practice" (2007, 190). Unequal access to sufficient and nutritious food was an issue for many of the families that I met over the course of my fieldwork. Equally, many state-maintained settings across England, such as Ladybird, are struggling to meet voluntary food guidelines, as they face financial constraints and cuts from their local councils.

These socio-economic variations, observable across the borough (and London), were noticeable also within Ladybird. At the time of my research, the school was state-maintained, and did not offer any places for fees, so parents who enrolled their children were from a range of socio-economic backgrounds – although prefer-ence for childcare places was given to families that received any form of state ben-efit. During the 2016–2017 academic year, 34% of children enrolled at the nursery were eligible for free school meals,[14] and a majority of families that accessed the services at the children's centre were in receipt of state benefits (between 55% and 65% of the approximately 450 active users at the centre, according to Ladybird's extended services manager).[15]

Poverty and inequality have severe consequences on the well-being of children (Child Poverty Action Group and Royal College of Paediatrics and Child Health (RCPCH) 2017). In 2015, the percentage of children living in out-of-work house-holds in the borough largely exceeded the inner/outer London average and the national average.[16] This alone suggests that high levels of child poverty exist in the borough, yet it is important to also note that, in the U.K., two-thirds of households where children live in relative poverty includes at least one adult who is employed (O'Connell, Knight, and Brannen 2019, 127). In England, as in other countries, children living in low-income households are more likely to experience food pov-erty and the related health issues that result from this (Child Poverty Action Group and Royal College of Paediatrics and Child Health (RCPCH) 2017, 6), including childhood obesity.

Researching childhood and the particularism of everyday life

Ladybird is minutes away from numerous public transport links and parallel to a bustling main road, yet it feels somewhat hidden away from the rest of the city. It is surrounded by three social housing estates and is adjacent to a quiet minor street. Aside from the busy morning drop-off and afternoon pick-up times, the area which surrounds the school is usually very quiet – the only noticeable sound is that of the children playing, laughing, or crying when they are in the school gardens at differ-ent points of the day.

Ladybird is divided into two sections (see Figure 0.1): walking in, to the right, is the nursery, which is comprised of three rooms and a separate, smaller room,

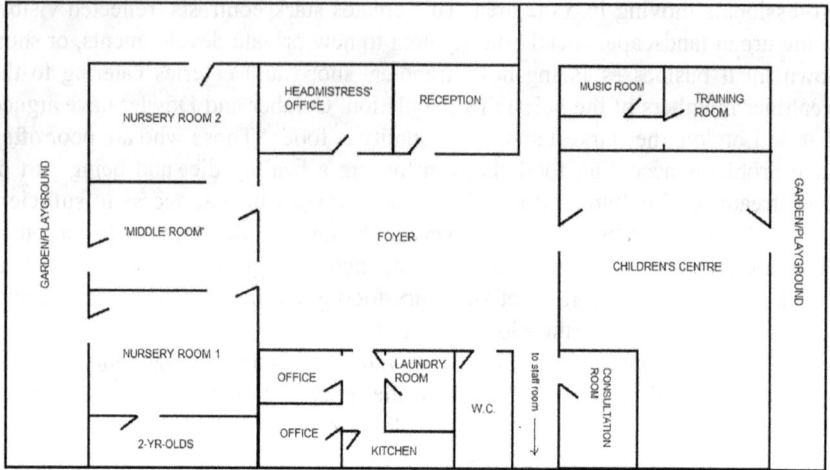

Figure 0.1 A floorplan of Ladybird Nursery and Children's Centre.
Image by the author.

which offers childcare for two-year-olds. The nursery rooms are laid out with a number of tables, on which different games and activities are set up each day for the children to choose from. In both Nursery Rooms 1 and 2 there are story book sections, where children can sit on a carpet when they read a book or are partaking in 'story time' with their teachers; each also have 'home corners,' comprised of a kitchen and living room set, and where costumes to play dressing up games are also available. The 'Middle Room' is dedicated to 'messy play': there is a sandbox here, and painting activities are usually carried out in this part of the nursery. Children eat lunch in each one of these rooms.

On the other hand, to the left of the main entrance, is the children's centre, where a variety of activities and services are provided, such as 'stay-and-play' sessions,[17] cooking and handcraft courses for parents, and breastfeeding and weaning support groups. The space is much smaller than the nursery, nonetheless, very similar activities are available to the children; here, too, is a home corner, different kinds of 'messy play,' dressing up, story books, building activities, as well as a 'baby corner,' where there is a variety of soft toys and books, rockers, and blankets. This is also, typically, the space where breastfeeding mothers go to when they feed their babies. Food here is served close to the kitchen's entrance; the open-plan kitchen is separated by a small dividing wall with a latch-door.

Ladybird is where I spent most of my time with children, practitioners, and families between 2016 and 2017. When not at the nursery or children's centre, I was in other settings within the borough where Ladybird is located, attending training about 'healthy eating' alongside some of the staff, or taking part in educational sessions delivered to families. Towards the end of my fieldwork, I also carried out interviews in families' homes.

Research with children

Over the year that I spent at Ladybird, I had the opportunity to partake in up to four mealtimes per day with the children: breakfast, lunch, afternoon snack time, and tea (or supper). In trying to understand what these different instances might have meant to them, and the relevance of food and mealtimes to daily life at school, I observed these moments, served food to the children, ate with them, talked with them about food and eating, and played with them in the 'kitchen corner.'

Reflecting on one's own position as a researcher, and the power relations between researcher and participants, is intrinsic to any ethnography, yet attention to this matter becomes even more important in the case of doing research with children. Two central concerns are that of gaining informed consent from child participants and ensuring their protection during the research process (Morrow and Richards 1996, 96).

There were several practical considerations related to gaining children's consent to participate in the research. As Morrow and Richards point out, "researchers usually obtain consent from a wide range of adult gatekeepers (parents, school teachers, head-teachers…and so on) […] In the U.K., consent is usually taken to mean consent from parents or those in 'loco parentis'" (1996, 94). However, the authors also argue that this is problematic given that it implies, to some degree, that children are not able to decide for themselves whether to take part in research. Aiming to resolve this tension, a distinction is made between consent and assent: although consent involves getting authorisation from an adult gatekeeper to involve a child in a research project, ultimately "the child assents or agrees to be a subject in the research" (ibid., 94). Acquiring consent is to be regarded as an ongoing negotiation between researcher and participants throughout the period of data collection (ibid., 101). Thus, as well as gaining parents' consent to carry out participant observation at Ladybird and to involve their children in child-centred research activities, I also always sought to be responsive to children's reactions and manners of engaging with me.

To do this, I followed Corsaro's 'reactive' approach (2011, 54) when conducting observation. I always asked the children if I could sit or play with them before setting out to do so. For visual activities, such as drawing and photo-elicitation, I would set up the materials on one of the tables in the classroom and wait for the children to approach me if they wanted to take part in an activity. Children initiated interactions by approaching my table and asking me what the activity was. If they wanted to partake after I explained the activity, they sat down with me and we would start the activity.

Throughout my time at Ladybird, I tried to remind children about my role in the setting whenever possible, as I did with the staff members I worked with and the parents I spoke with. What I found most straightforward to articulate to children was that I was writing a book about the food they liked, and that I was interested in finding out what they ate in school and at home, which is why I spent time with them at Ladybird, particularly when they had their mealtimes. Following Mandell's idea of adopting the 'least adult role' (1988; see also Warming 2005), children knew from the outset that I was not a teacher, and I tried to further emphasise this by doing things other adults would not do, such as dressing up in costume if they wanted me to partake in dress-up games, or giving them my badge[18] to play with. This is in line with Warming's suggestion that to distinguish oneself as an 'atypical adult' within a childcare setting, we must relinquish some of our authority and allow for role reversal to occur when possible (2005, 59). In practice, this was of course a delicate terrain to navigate, since (due to my volunteering in the setting) children often saw me in roles that other staff members also fulfilled. Similarly, due to the frequent need to manage everyday risks related to childcare (for example, having to intervene if children had any conflicts with each other, or helping children in the playground if they got hurt), I was not always able to forgo the authoritative position other adults occupied.

In addition to traditional ethnographic approaches, I also used child-centred methods in my research, particularly visual methods (photo-elicitation, drawing activities, and story-telling). I drew predominantly from the work of Punch (2002a) and O'Connell (2013) to develop the different visual activities that I conducted with child participants. Punch argues that:

> The advantages of using drawing with children is that it can be creative, fun and encourage children to be more actively involved in the research. The use of drawing gives children time to think about what they wish to portray. The image can be changed and added to, which gives children more control over their form of expression, unlike an interview situation where responses tend to be quicker and more immediate.
>
> (2002a, 331)

In a mixed methods study of family food practices, O'Connell employed a range of qualitative visual methods, which included: "timelines; photographic vignettes; participant generated photoelicitation; a shopping trolley activity [and] a paper plate exercise" (2013, 35). Quoting Bagnoli (2009), and similarly to Punch (2002a), O'Connell suggests that, "visual approaches generate additional insights over and 'beyond the standard interview'" (2013, 42), as well as allowing participants to "re-represent the world in a way that makes it more accessible to the beholder than words alone" (ibid.).

I used three visual activities with child participants. First, a paper plate activity, where I gave children two plates to draw on. On one of them I asked children to draw their favourite foods to eat at home, on another what they liked to eat at school. We would then talk about the drawings, often linking to ongoing conversations we had on when, with whom, and in which situations they would have these meals. Second, I used a photo-elicitation activity to also have conversations with children about food, eating at home, and eating at Ladybird. I used a cardboard box[19] decorated with colourful paper and different images of foods, and I invited children to open the box and choose the images they wanted to talk about.

The third visual method I used was a child-led free-drawing activity. I used photographic vignettes as conversation prompts but also as aids for the free-drawing exercise. In addition to photographs, I also used a children's picture book titled *1000 Things to Eat* (Wood and Dyson 2015), which depicts a variety of food types and dishes from around the world, many of which were recognisable to children, and which also provided some starting points both for conversation topics and the drawings children made.

It is worth mentioning, nonetheless, that doing research with children should not be viewed as 'entertaining,' or the methods seen as 'simple,' as this can be patronising to participants or minimise their contributions (Punch 2002a, 329–30). Drawing from James et al. (1997), this matter was managed in this project by thinking about different methods of data gathering not as 'child friendly,' but as child-centred, that is, addressed to the competencies of the participants.

Research with practitioners

Creating rapport with some of the early years practitioners at Ladybird took a couple of months, since my ambiguous position as researcher and volunteer was unprecedented at the setting. At times it was difficult to understand how much I should be helping out, particularly at the children's centre where my duties were less well-defined than when I assisted staff during lunchtime at the nursery. Learning to navigate work-place politics and not to step on anyone's toes was a challenge, yet re-learning how to do certain tasks, in a manner that was appropriate to the context I was in, was also a difficult process, and the mistakes that I occasionally made felt like big setbacks at the beginning.

An early example of this was being asked to cut up fruit for snacks at the children's centre for the first time. I knew the apples I was given should probably not be served in small pieces, to avoid creating a choking hazard, so I diced them into chunky cubes. However, even with this consideration in mind, I did not carry out the task correctly. Joyce, the lead early years practitioner at the children's centre, kindly but firmly instructed me to cut apples and pears in a 'half-moon' shape in the future, so that children could hold them in their hands easily. Cutting the apple into thinner slices also meant that we could get more servings out of one piece of fruit, which was very important given that fresh fruit was a limited resource at the children's centre. This instance might seem trite, but it is representative of the amount of energy, attention, and dedication childcare work requires.

Despite the initial challenges, after a few weeks, and certainly within two months or so of me being there, it started to feel like I had become part of daily life at Ladybird. I was still 'other' but had a clearer set of roles and closer relationships with many of the staff. As with child participants, there were many occasions in which I had the opportunity to remind adults of my capacity as researcher in the setting, and this was also evident to them because of things like my occasional, quick note-taking while going about daily duties, or the conversations they heard me have with parents. Soon, some of the staff began to actively contribute to my research activities, either by introducing me to families they thought might want to take part in home interviews, by inviting me along to some of the food-related training activities around the borough (which they had to attend), or by saving flyers or other hard copies of information they thought would be useful for me to have. As time went by, people began to open up more about their views on children's food, what they thought about their roles when feeding children, and their rationale for reaching out to some parents (but not others) to share information and advice about food.

Being a childcare worker of sorts was also very much part of my research process, and what enabled me to arrive at many of my findings, even if there were times in which I was immersed in the field as just a researcher (like during child-centred activities) and my role as an anthropologist was thus a lot more obvious. There were different ways in which I managed this 'double identity.' For example, at times when I felt that particularly sensitive topics had been discussed with me, I would ask people whether they were comfortable with me using what they had shared in my research or not, and often this would lead to even more interesting discussions that participants felt were important for me to include in my work.

I often asked participants if *they* had any questions for me. People wanted to know about my own eating practices, or were interested to know about my personal life (where I was from, whether one day I also wanted a family, what it is like to be a researcher). I felt this allowed me to better manage the power dynamics between researcher and participants, as it was a way to acknowledge that I was not the only one observing, but that I was being observed as well, and that I had to navigate access, and earn children's and adults' trust, at all times.

Research with parents

I met and talked with parents on many occasions during my time at Ladybird, but primarily during 'stay and play' sessions at the children's centre. As with children and staff, I spent several months just getting acquainted with people. Some parents were regular visitors to the centre, others only came for brief periods of time, or sporadically. These sessions were a good way to meet families, since (unlike at the nursery), parents and other carers would stay with their children at the setting, and socialise with one another and staff, whilst the children played. The children's centre was also where parents and children attended educational activities, such as arts and crafts courses and cooking classes. I also became well-acquainted with parents of children who attended 'tea-club' in the afternoons, as their pick-up time was usually less rushed and chaotic than the main drop-off and pick-up routine at the nursery.

Similarly to my relationship with early years practitioners, it took a couple of months before I felt like the parents and I had established meaningful rapport. Conversations with them about my research and role(s) at Ladybird were ongoing throughout the time that I spent conducting fieldwork. With parents, one of the main obstacles was making sure that they did not misunderstand my area of research, as in the beginning they assumed that I was a medical professional and that my research was about 'improving' children's diets. In the beginning, I was sometimes asked for nutritional advice, and sometimes I was also asked for help if children were 'fussy eaters.' To these questions I always responded by saying that, having no medical background, I was not in a position to give such advice. I explained that my interest was in understanding children's everyday lives at the nursery, particularly how they interacted with each other and adults during mealtimes: "the social aspect of food and eating," I usually said. Like with the staff, as time went on, some of the parents started to contribute to my research in their own way, by spontaneously coming up to me to talk about things they thought I might find interesting (perhaps something their child had said or done at home), about something they had cooked for their family, or their experiences with health professionals or other encounters with official actors.

One barrier I thought I might face in conducting research with parents is the fact that I do not have any children myself, and thus that I might ask very obvious (or wrong) questions. Yet, whilst adding to my 'outsider' position, this helped me to not take things for granted: everything that I noticed was new and interesting to me. Parents did not view my inexperience as an obstacle when speaking to me, but rather as an opportunity to explain things to me in detail.

Finally, whilst I have been speaking in general terms of 'parents' and 'early years practitioners,' it is important to note that the majority of adult participants I spoke with were women. The question of gender in the context of carework and foodwork will be explored at length in Chapters 4 and 6. A lack of male voices in this book, whilst unintentional, very much reflects that childcare (domestic and otherwise) and feeding children are still predominantly female domains.

Chapter outline

Each chapter in this book will unpack the overarching theme of universalism versus particularism from a different angle, relying on the various perspectives of the people I encountered in the year that I spent at Ladybird.

In Chapter 1, I provide an analysis of the policy discourses that shaped practices on the ground by examining four secondary sources using Bacchi and Goodwin's 'What's the Problem Represented to be?' (WPR) approach (2016). Specifically, the chapter unpacks official discourses around childhood obesity and sugar intake, and questions the prominence that lack of knowledge and skills, insufficient early intervention, and 'inadequate parenting' have been given as reasons for these 'problems' to persist. This discussion provides the basis needed to later explore the tensions that these universal understandings created in the particular, daily interactions that took place at Ladybird and in participants' homes. Chapter 2 unpacks some of the interactions between the state and food industry, showing the contradictions that can arise when marketed food products are included in policy and public health encounters. The themes of responsibility and individual accountability are unpacked in these two chapters to show how these notions are operationalised at the macro-level.

Chapter 3 builds on the analysis presented in Chapters 1 and 2 to explore Ladybird staff members' feeding practices. I ask what were the aims that adults pursued when feeding children at the setting, and how these were shaped by (and in tension with) official discourses, as well as the different regulations and guidelines that early years providers are expected to follow. I argue that food and mealtimes were often used as 'pedagogical tools' by staff members at Ladybird, to teach children about 'healthy' eating, table manners, and to address the issue of 'fussy eating.' Parallel to these overarching 'pedagogical' aims, this chapter explores the practical dimension of feeding children at Ladybird, as well as the contradictions that might emerge when staff needed to balance their personal ethics of care with the logistical and bureaucratic aspects of institutional feeding. I argue that feeding children in an institutional context poses some social and emotional limits on early years practitioners, creating a contrast between their personal ethics of care and the practical aspect of their work.

Chapter 4 turns to children's eating practices at Ladybird, unpacking their experiences from their own points of view. Following Corsaro's work on 'interpretive reproduction' (2011), this section asks how children create self- and peer-group identities through food and eating practices. Focusing on play behaviour, humour, and role reversal, I explore the different interactions through which group unity was achieved among children. By considering children's different forms of communication as 'idioms of childhood' (Nolas, Aruldoss, and Varvantakis 2018), this chapter also examines what children considered meaningful about food and mealtimes. I will show that children represented (and performed) food and mealtimes as channels through which to express care, enact authority, and communicate their knowledge about food and social relationships. Finally, I explore how children negotiated power relations with school staff during mealtimes. I suggest that Bakhtin's 'dialogic' (1986) may complement Corsaro's notions about 'interpretive reproduction' (2011), adding to our understanding of how children's knowledge and sense of self is produced co-relationally, through their engagement with the multiple social worlds that they inhabit.

Chapter 5 explores Ladybird's role as a provider of 'extended' (welfare) services to 'target families.' Building on the notion of food as a 'pedagogical tool,' and linking to the idea that early years settings have historically been perceived as sites within which perceived deficiencies in the domestic sphere can be rectified, I will examine how three different family interventions were promoted and operationalised on the ground by a number of actors. In this chapter, I empirically assess how the official discourses that I unpacked in Chapter 1 unfold in the lives of 'target groups,' and how the assumptions underlying these discourses shape the interactions between those who promote interventions, and the families that partake in them. Parallel to this, I examine how the Mixed Economy of Welfare (MEW) (Powell 2014) functions in practice. In exploring the contradictions and arbitrariness inherent in food and family interventions, I highlight the challenges that parents face when feeding their children, which are often not in line with the official assumptions that guide food, public health, and family intervention policies.

Using a gender lens (Cairns and Johnston 2015), the final chapter of this book will centre on mothers' accounts of feeding their children. In contrast to the discussion on responsibility and individual accountability presented in Chapter 1, Chapter 6 explores how the themes of responsibility and control emerged on the micro-level in the semi-structured interviews that I conducted with three mothers. Returning to Foucault's conceptualisation of governmentality as "diffuse" (Foucault 1991;

Lupton 1995, 9), I will examine women's accounts of self-scrutiny, and of trying to maintain control of their children's eating. Much of the available literature on this topic, and some of what participants related to me, emphasise that children's acts of resistance during mealtimes are often experienced as 'defeats' by mothers, focusing on the oppressive quality that foodwork can often take in women's lives. In the final section of this chapter, I assess these claims, yet aim to simultaneously provide a counter-narrative by showing that, when at school, children also reproduced some of the norms and practices that their mothers promoted at home. Conversely, some of the practices children brought from the school into the home were well-received by parents. Drawing from Bakhtin (1986), I will show that it is not only children who respond to and reinterpret their parents' views on food and eating, but it is also adults who react to children's newly acquired preferences. I argue that it is thus important to analyse mothers' feeding as part of the mutualistic and caring production of norms and practices that adults and children engage in together. By examining how children reinterpret norms and behaviours from the home and school environments, bringing them into each context, the 'back and forth' interaction between different realms is once again brought to light. Throughout the book, the particularistic theme of childhood becomes the lens through which the universalism of policy and bureaucracy is problematised and challenged.

Notes

1 The name of the setting where I carried out my research has been changed to protect participants' anonymity.

2 I use inverted commas here, and throughout the book, when assigning any kind of value-laden adjective to food. As it will become clear throughout the book, 'healthy food' can mean different things to different people, and even official guidelines (which are thought of as neutral and objective) can be blurry.

3 A brand of small-sized, hard candy, available in a number of flavours.

4 The cooking classes always began with an informal chat, during which sliced fruit was available as a snack to the participants.

5 Foucault defines the emergence of biopower in the 18th century as replacing the "old power of death that symbolized sovereign power" with "numerous and diverse techniques for achieving the subjugation of bodies and the control of populations" (1978, 139–40), for instance, through public health policy.

6 It is important to note that these are not phenomena confined to the U.K.; women's (and children's) lack of political leverage is historically and geographically pervasive (Lister 2003, 68–73).

7 A childminder is a person who looks after children in their own home.

8 "You can usually get 30 hours free childcare if you (and your partner, if you have one) are: in work, on sick leave or annual leave, on parental, maternity or adoption leave. If you're on parental leave, you cannot apply for the child you're on leave for." Available from: https://www.gov.uk/30-hours-free-childcare [Accessed 26/6/2019].

9 This policy was first proposed under former (Conservative) Prime Minister David Cameron. In a January 2016 speech he gave on "improving life chances," he stated that, "because the evidence shows that families where only one parent is in work are more at risk of poverty we are going to back all those who want to work. That's why our offer for working parents – of 30 hours a week of free childcare for 3 and 4 year olds – is so important" (Cameron 2016).

10 "The Childcare Bill is delivering the government's election manifesto commitment to giving families where parents are working an entitlement to 30 hours of free childcare for their three- and four-year olds. The Childcare Bill was introduced to the House of Lords on 1 June 2015. This statement is made available to the House of Lords to aid Peers in their scrutiny of the Childcare Bill ahead of Report stage" (Department for Education 2015, 3).

11 Professionalism is also a contested domain in feminist texts dealing with care. On one hand, increasing professionalization of the care workforce serves to counteract essentialist notions of caregiving as an innate practice that does not require formal training (Tronto 2013, 7–8), and also opposes the undervalued (and often exploitative) status that carework currently holds in most societies. On the other, some authors also emphasise that a move towards standardisation and monetisation of caregiving can undermine the emotional/intrapersonal element that carework necessarily entails (Abel and Nelson 1990, 5–6).

12 Drawing from Ariès' premise that children – perceived as "too fragile" to partake in the adult world – simply "did not count" in pre-16th and 17th century society (Ariès 1962, 128).

13 The categories included: Bangladeshi, Black – Congolese, Black – Ghanaian, Black – Nigerian, Black – Sierra Leonean, Chinese, Indian, Latin/South/Central American, Turkish, Vietnamese, White, White and Black African, White – Eastern European, White – English, White – Other, White – Western European, Any Other Asian Background, Any Other Black Background, Any Other Mixed Background.

14 To be eligible for free school meals at the nursery, one or more parent in a household must be receiving one of the following benefits: income support, income based Job Seekers Allowance, income related Employment and Support Allowance, NASS (Asylum) support, Child Tax Credit, Working Tax Credit, or Universal Credit [information available from Ladybird Nursery website].

15 This has changed since the year in which I conducted fieldwork, following the launch of the 30-hours free childcare allowance for working parents discussed earlier.

16 London Borough Profiles. Available from: https://londondatastore-upload.s3.amazonaws.com/instant-atlas/borough-profiles/atlas.html.

17 Sessions for infants to play and interact with each other, in the company of their parents or other carers.

18 The badge was necessary to open doors within the school, and all staff members and volunteers had to carry one around their necks. My badge also contributed to distinguishing me from other adults as it did not have a photograph of me on it, a point which the children often brought up and which gave me an opportunity to remind them about my role at Ladybird.

19 Similarly to Punch's 'secret box' technique in conducting qualitative research with teenagers (Punch 2002b).

References

Abel, Emily K., and Margaret K. Nelson. 1990. 'Circles of Care: An Introductory Essay'. In *Circles of Care: Work and Identity in Women's Life*, edited by Emily K. Abel and Margaret K. Nelson, 4–34. New York: State University of New York Press.

Akresh, Ilana Redstone. 2007. 'Dietary Assimilation and Health among Hispanic Immigrants to the United States'. *Journal of Health and Social Behavior* 48 (4): 404–17.

Alexander, Claire. 2011. 'Making Bengali Brick Lane: Claiming and Contesting Space in East London: Making Bengali Brick Lane'. *The British Journal of Sociology* 62 (2): 201–20. https://doi.org/10.1111/j.1468-4446.2011.01361.x.

Ariès, Philippe. 1962. *Centuries of Childhood: A Social History of Family Life*. New York: Vintage Books.

Bacchi, Carol, and Susan Goodwin. 2016. *Poststructural Policy Analysis: A Guide to Practice*. New York: Palgrave Macmillan.

Back, Les, and Shamser Sinha. 2018. *Migrant City*. London: Routledge.

Bagnoli, A. 2009. 'Beyond the Standard Interview: The Use of Graphic Elicitation and Arts-Based Methods'. *Qualitative Research* 9 (5): 547–70.

Bakhtin, Mikhail. 1981. *The Dialogic Imagination: Four Essays*. Austin: University of Texas Press.

———. 1986. *Speech Genres and Other Late Essays*. Austin: University of Texas Press.

Berg, Mette Louise, and Nando Sigona. 2013. 'Ethnography, Diversity and Urban Space'. *Identities* 20 (4): 347–60. https://doi.org/10.1080/1070289X.2013.822382.

Bluebond-Langner, Myra, and Jill E. Korbin. 2007. 'Challenges and Opportunities in the Anthropology of Childhoods: An Introduction to "Children, Childhoods, and Childhood Studies"'. *American Anthropologist* 109 (2): 241–46. https://doi.org/10.1525/aa.2007.109.2.241.

Boni, Zofia. 2017. 'It's Safe: Food as a Way of Expression for Children in Warsaw'. *Children's Geographies*, May, 1–12. https://doi.org/10.1080/14733285.2017.1319045.

———. 2023. *Feeding Anxieties: The Politics of Children's Food in Poland*. Vol. 6. New Anthropologies of Europe: Perspectives and Provocations. New York and Oxford: Berghahn Books.

Butler, Tim, Chris Hamnett, and Mark Ramsden. 2008. 'Inward and Upward: Marking Out Social Class Change in London, 1981–2001'. *Urban Studies* 45 (1): 67–88. https://doi.org/10.1177/0042098007085102.

Cairns, Kate, and Johnston, Josée. 2015. *Food and Femininity*. New York: Bloomsbury.

Cameron, David. 2016. 'Prime Minister's Speech on Life Chances'. GOV.UK. https://www.gov.uk/government/speeches/prime-ministers-speech-on-life-chances.

Caraher, Martin, and Elizabeth Dowler. 2007. 'Food Projects in London: Lessons for Policy and Practice—A Hidden Sector and the Need for "More Unhealthy Puddings… Sometimes"'. *Health Education Journal* 66 (2): 188–205.

Child Poverty Action Group and Royal College of Paediatrics and Child Health (RCPCH). 2017. 'Poverty and Child Health: Views from the Frontline'. London: Child Poverty Action Group. http://www.cpag.org.uk/sites/default/files/pdf%20RCPCH.pdf.

Chowbey, Punita, and Deborah Harrop. 2016. 'Healthy Eating in UK Minority Ethnic Households: Influences and Way Forward'. London: Race Equality Foundation. http://www.better-health.org.uk/sites/default/files/briefings/downloads/Better%20Health%2042%20-%20Healthy%20Eating%20[final].pdf.

Clarke, Karen. 2006. 'Childhood, Parenting and Early Intervention: A Critical Examination of the Sure Start National Programme'. *Critical Social Policy* 26 (4): 699–721. https://doi.org/10.1177/0261018306068470.

Cooper, Elizabeth Elliott. 2013. 'Does Child Food Exist for Rural Malays? A Mixed Methods Approach to Food and Identity'. *Food and Foodways* 21 (3): 211–35. https://doi.org/10.1080/07409710.2013.821298.

Corsaro, William. 2005. 'Collective Action and Agency in Young Children's Peer Culture'. In *Studies in Modern Childhood: Society, Agency, Culture*, edited by Jens Qvortrup, 231–47. Basingstoke: Palgrave Macmillan.

———. 2011. *The Sociology of Childhood*. London: SAGE Publications.

Coveney, John. 2000. 'The Governmentality of Modern Nutrition'. In *Food, Morals and Meaning: The Pleasure and Anxiety of Eating*, 15–24. London: Routledge.

Cox, Rachael, Ruth Emond, Samantha Punch, Ian McIntosh, Kate Hall, Angela Simpson, and Helen Skouteris. 2017. '"It's Not as Easy as Saying, 'Just Get Them to Eat More

Veggies'": Exploring Healthy Eating in Residential Care in Australia'. *Appetite* 117 (October): 275–83. https://doi.org/10.1016/j.appet.2017.07.004.

DeLoache, Judy, and Alma Gottlieb, eds. 2000. *A World of Babies: Imagined Childcare Guides for Seven Societies*. Cambridge: Cambridge University Press.

Department for Communities and Local Government. 2015. 'English Indices of Deprivation 2015'. London: The Department for Communities and Local Government. https://assets.publishing.service.gov.uk/government/uploads/system/uploads/attachment_data/file/465791/English_Indices_of_Deprivation_2015_-_Statistical_Release.pdf.

———. 2019. 'The English Indices of Deprivation 2019'. London: The Department for Communities and Local Government. https://assets.publishing.service.gov.uk/government/uploads/system/uploads/attachment_data/file/835115/IoD2019_Statistical_Release.pdf.

Department for Education. 2015. 'Chilcare Bill: Policy Statement'. https://www.gov.uk/government/uploads/system/uploads/attachment_data/file/465446/Childcare_Bill_Policy_statement.pdf.

———. 2016. 'Provision for Children under Five Years of Age in England, January 2016'. London: Department for Education. https://assets.publishing.service.gov.uk/government/uploads/system/uploads/attachment_data/file/532575/SFR23_2016_Text.pdf.

———. 2017. 'Statutory Framework for the Early Years Foundation Stage: Setting the Standards for Learning, Development and Care for Children from Birth to Five'. London: Department for Education. https://assets.publishing.service.gov.uk/government/uploads/system/uploads/attachment_data/file/596629/EYFS_STATUTORY_FRAMEWORK_2017.pdf.Dorrer, Nika, Ian McIntosh, Samantha Punch, and Ruth Emond. 2010. 'Children and Food Practices in Residential Care: Ambivalence in the "Institutional" Home'. *Children's Geographies* 8 (3): 247–59. https://doi.org/10.1080/14733285.2010.494863.

Edminston, Daniel. 2018. *Welfare, Inequality and Social Citizenship: Deprivation and Affluence in Austerity Britain*. Bristol: Policy Press.

Evans, John, Laura De Pian, Emma Rich, and Brian Davies. 2011. 'Health Imperatives, Policy and the Corporeal Device: Schools, Subjectivity and Children's Health'. *Policy Futures in Education* 9 (3): 328–40. https://doi.org/10.2304/pfie.2011.9.3.328.

Foucault, Michel. 1978. *The History of Sexuality, Vol. 1: An Introduction*. New York: Pantheon Books.

———. 1988. 'Technologies of the Self'. In *Technologies of the Self: A Seminar with Michel Foucault*, edited by Luther H. Martin, Huck Gutman, and Patrick H. Hutton, 16–49. London: Tavistock Publications Ltd.

———. 1991. 'Governmentality'. In *The Foucault Effect: Studies in Governmentality, with Two Lectures by and an Interview with Michel Foucault*, edited by Graham Burchell, Colin Gordon, and Peter Miller. Chicago: University of Chicago Press. 87-104.

Gibson, Megan, Felicity McArdle, and Caroline Hatcher. 2015. 'Governing Child Care in Neoliberal Times: Discursive Constructions of Children as Economic Units and Early Childhood Educators as Investment Brokers'. *Global Studies of Childhood* 5 (3): 322–32. https://doi.org/10.1177/2043610615597149.

Goodwill, Robert, and Robert Goodwill. 2017. 'Benefits of 30 Hours Confirmed as Free Childcare Places Soar'. GOV.UK. 18 July 2017. https://www.gov.uk/government/news/benefits-of-30-hours-confirmed-as-free-childcare-places-soar.

Gottlieb, Alma. 1998. 'Do Infants Have Religion? The Spiritual Lives of Beng Babies'. *American Anthropologist* 100 (1): 122–35.

———. 2004. *The Afterlife Is Where We Come from: The Culture of Infancy in West Africa*. Chicago: University of Chicago Press.

Gupta, Akhil. 2012. *Red Tape Bureaucracy, Structural Violence, and Poverty in India.* Durham: Duke University Press.

Halkier, Bente, and Iben Jensen. 2011. 'Doing "Healthier" Food in Everyday Life? A Qualitative Study of How Pakistani Danes Handle Nutritional Communication'. *Critical Public Health* 21 (4): 471–83. https://doi.org/10.1080/09581596.2011.594873.

Hall, Suzanne. 2008. 'Narrating the City: Diverse Spaces of Urban Change, South London'. *Open House International* 33 (2): 10–17.

Hlaimi, Stephane. 2021. 'The Effects of Brexit and Covid-19 on Food Inflation in the United Kingdom', December. https://doi.org/10.5281/ZENODO.5791132.

James, Allison, and Alan Prout. 1997. *Constructing and Reconstructing Childhood: Contemporary Issues in the Sociological Study of Childhood.* London: Falmer Press.

Lancy, David F. 2008. *The Anthropology of Childhood: Cherubs, Chattel, Changelings.* Cambridge: Cambridge University Press.

Lang, Tim. 2019. 'No-Deal Food Planning in UK Brexit'. *The Lancet*, August. https://doi.org/10.1016/S0140-6736(19)31769-6.

Lang, Tim, Erik Millstone, Tony Lewis, and Terry Marsden. 2018. 'Feeding Britain: Food Security after Brexit'. London: Food Research Collaboration. http://foodresearch.org.uk/publications/feeding-britain-food-security-after-brexit/.

Leahy, Deana. 2014. 'Assembling a Health[y] Subject: Risky and Shameful Pedagogies in Health Education'. *Critical Public Health* 24 (2): 171–81. https://doi.org/10.1080/09581596.2013.871504.

Leahy, Deana, and Jan Wright. 2016. 'Governing Food Choices: A Critical Analysis of School Food Pedagogies and Young People's Responses in Contemporary Times'. *Cambridge Journal of Education* 46 (2): 233–46. https://doi.org/10.1080/0305764X.2015.1118440.

Lee, Ellie, Jennie Bristow, Charlotte Faircloth, and Jan Macvarish. 2014. *Parenting Culture Studies.* Basingstoke: Palgrave Macmillan.

Lewis, J. 2013. 'Continuity and Change in English Childcare Policy 1960-2000'. *Social Politics: International Studies in Gender, State & Society* 20 (3): 358–86. https://doi.org/10.1093/sp/jxt013.

Lister, Ruth. 2003. *Citizisenship: Feminist Perspectives.* London: Palgrave Macmillan.

Loopstra, R., A. Reeves, D. Taylor-Robinson, B. Barr, M. McKee, and D. Stuckler. 2015. 'Austerity, Sanctions, and the Rise of Food Banks in the UK'. *BMJ* 350 (apr08 9): h1775. https://doi.org/10.1136/bmj.h1775.

Lupton, Deborah. 1995. *The Imperative of Health: Public Health and the Regulated Body.* London: SAGE Publications.

———. 1996. *Food, the Body and the Self.* London: SAGE Publications.

Maher, JaneMaree, Suzanne Fraser, and Jo Lindsay. 2010. 'Between Provisioning and Consuming?: Children, Mothers and "Childhood Obesity"'. *Health Sociology Review* 19 (3): 304–16.

Maher, JaneMaree, Suzanne Fraser, and Jan Wright. 2010. 'Framing the Mother: Childhood Obesity, Maternal Responsibility and Care'. *Journal of Gender Studies* 19 (3): 233–47. https://doi.org/10.1080/09589231003696037.

Mannion, Greg. 2018. 'Intergenerational Education and Learning: We Are in a New Place'. In *Families, Intergenerationality, and Peer Group Relations,* edited by Samantha Punch, Robert M. Vanderbeck and Tracey Skelton. Singapore: Springer Nature.

Matos Viegas, Susana de. 2003. 'Eating with Your Favourite Mother: Time and Sociality in a Brazilian Amerindian Community'. *Journal of the Royal Anthropological Institute* 9 (1): 21–37.

Mayall, Berry. 2006. 'Values and Assumptions Underpinning Policy for Children and Young People in England'. *Children's Geographies* 4 (1): 9–17. https://doi.org/10.1080/14733280600576923.

Mayerfeld Bell, Michael. 1998. 'Culture as Dialogue'. In *Bakhtin and the Human Sciences: No Last Words*, edited by Michael Mayerfeld Bell and Michael Gardiner, 49–62. London: SAGE Publications.

McIntosh, Ian, Samantha Punch, Ruth Emond, Kirsi Pauliina Kallio, Sarah Mills, and Tracey Skelton. 2015. 'Creating Spaces to Care: Children's Rights and Food Practices in Residential Care'. In *Politics, Citizenship and Rights*. Vol. 7. Springer Major Reference Work in Geographies of Children and Young People. Singapore: Springer.

McKenzie, Lisa. 2015. *Getting by: Estates, Class and Culture in Austerity Britain*. Bristol: Policy Press.

Mead, Margaret. 1928. *Coming of Age in Samoa : A Psychological Study of Primitive Youth for Western Civilisation*. New York: W. Morrow & Company.

Michel, S. 2002. 'Afterword: Dilemmas of Childcare'. In *Child Care Policy at the Crossroads. Gender and Welfare State Restructuring*, edited by R. Mahon and S. Michel. New York: Routlegde.

Millstone, Erik, Tim Lang, and Terry Marsden. 2019. 'Food Brexit and Chlorinated Chicken: A Microcosm of Wider Food Problems'. *The Political Quarterly* 90 (4): 645–53. https://doi.org/10.1111/1467-923X.12780.

Mol, Annemarie. 2008. *The Logic of Care: Health and the Problem of Patient Choice*. London: Routledge.

Montgomery, Heather. 2009. *An Introduction to Childhood: Anthropological Perspectives on Children's Lives*. Oxford: Wiley-Blackwell.

Morrow, Virginia and Martin Richards. 1996. 'The Ethics of Social Research with Children: An Overview'. *Children & Society*, 10: 90–105. https://doi.org/10.1111/j.1099-0860.1996.tb00461.x

Moss, Peter. 2012. 'Poor, Consumer, Citizen? What Image of the Parent in England?' *Rivista Italiana Di Educazione Familiare* 1: 63–78.

———. 2015. 'There Are Alternatives! Contestation and Hope in Early Childhood Education'. *Global Studies of Childhood* 5 (3): 226–38. https://doi.org/10.1177/2043610615597130.

Moss, Peter, and Pat Petrie. 2000. *From Children's Services to Children's Spaces*. London: Routledge/Falmer.

Mosse, David. 2005. *Cultivating Development: An Ethnography of Aid Policy and Practice*. London: Pluto Press.

Nielsen, Annette, Alan Krasnik, and Lotte Holm. 2013. 'Ethnicity and Children's Diets: The Practices and Perceptions of Mothers in Two Minority Ethnic Groups in Denmark'. *Mother & Child Nutrition* 11 (4): 948–61.

Nolas, Sevasti-Melissa, Vinnarasan Aruldoss, and Christos Varvantakis. 2018. 'Learning to Listen: Exploring the Idioms of Childhood'. *Sociological Research Online*, 24 (3): 1–20.

O'Connell, Rebecca. 2013. 'The Use of Visual Methods with Children in a Mixed Methods Study of Family Food Practices'. *International Journal of Social Research Methodology* 16 (1): 31–46. https://doi.org/10.1080/13645579.2011.647517.

O'Connell, Rebecca, and Julia Brannen. 2016. *Food, Families and Work*. London: Bloomsbury.

O'Connell, Rebecca, Abigail Knight, and Julia Brannen. 2019. *Living Hand to Mouth: Children and Food in Low-Income Families*. London: Child Poverty Action Group.

Peck, Jamie, and Nik Theodore. 2012. 'Reanimating Neoliberalism: Process Geographies of Neoliberalisation'. *Social Anthropology* 20 (2): 177–85. https://doi.org/10.1111/j.1469-8676.2012.00194.x.

Penn, Helen. 2007. 'Childcare Market Management: How the United Kingdom Government Has Reshaped Its Role in Developing Early Childhood Education and Care'. *Contemporary Issues in Early Childhood* 8 (3): 192–207. https://doi.org/10.2304/ciec.2007.8.3.192.

———. 2011. 'Policy Rationales for Early Childhood Services'. *International Journal of Child Care and Education Policy* 5 (1): 1–16. https://doi.org/10.1007/2288-6729-5-1-1.

Petherick, LeAnne. 2015. 'Shaping the Child as a Healthy Child: Health Surveillance, Schools, and Biopedagogies'. *Cultural Studies? Critical Methodologies* 15 (5): 361–70.

Pike, Jo. 2008. 'Foucault, Space and Primary School Dining Rooms'. *Children's Geographies* 6 (4): 413–22.

———.2010. '"I don't have to listen to you! You're just a dinner lady!": Power and Resistance at Lunchtimes in Primary Schools'. *Children's Geographies* 8 (3): 275–87.

Pike, Jo, and Deana Leahy. 2012. 'School Food and the Pedagogies of Parenting'. *Australian Journal of Adult Learning* 52 (3): 434.

Platt, Lucinda. 2007. 'Child Poverty, Employment and Ethnicity in the UK: The Role and Limitations of Policy'. *European Societies* 9 (2): 175–99. https://doi.org/10.1080/14616690701217809.

Powell, Martin. 2014. *Understanding the Mixed Economy of Welfare*. Bristol: The Policy Press.

Power, Michael. 1999. *The Audit Society: Rituals of Verification*. Oxford: Oxford University Press.

Pre-school Learning Alliance. 2017. 'Sector Views on Early Years Funding and the 30-Hour Offer'. London: Early Years Alliance. https://www.eyalliance.org.uk/sites/default/files/30-hour_and_funding_survey_-_pre-school_learning_alliance.pdf.

Punch, Samantha. 2002a. 'RESEARCH WITH CHILDREN: The Same or Different from Research with Adults?' *Childhood* 9 (3): 321–41.

———. 2002b. 'Interviewing Strategies with Young People: The "Secret Box", Stimulus Material and Task-Based Activities'. *Children & Society* 16 (1): 45–56. https://doi.org/10.1002/chi.685.Punch, Samantha, Ian McIntosh, and Ruth Emond. 2012. '"You Have a Right to Be Nourished and Fed, but Do I Have a Right to Make Sure You Eat Your Food?": Children's Rights and Food Practices in Residential Care'. *The International Journal of Human Rights* 16 (8): 1250–62. https://doi.org/10.1080/13642987.2012.728858.

Punch, S., & McIntosh, I. (2014). 'Food is a funny thing within residential child care': Intergenerational relationships and food practices in residential care. Childhood, 21(1), 72–86. https://doi.org/10.1177/0907568213481814

Punch, Samantha and Robert M. Vanderbeck. 2018. 'Families, Intergenerationality, and Peer Group Relations: Introduction'. In *Families, Intergenerationality, and Peer Group Relations*, edited by Samantha Punch, Robert M. Vanderbeck and Tracey Skelton. Singapore: Springer Nature.

Qvortrup, Jens. 2005. 'Varieties of Childhood'. In *Studies in Modern Childhood: Society, Agency, Culture*, edited by Jens Qvortrup, 1–20. Basingstoke: Palgrave Macmillan.

———. 2011. 'Childhood as a Structural Form'. In *The Palgrave Handbook of Childhood Studies*, edited by Jens Qvortrup, William Corsaro, and Michael-Sebastian Honing, 21–33. Basingstoke: Palgrave Macmillan.

Randall, Vicky. 2000. *The Politics of Child Daycare in Britain*. Oxford: Oxford University Press.

———. 2002. 'Child Care in Britain, or, How Do You Restructure Nothing?' In *Child Care Policy at the Crossroads. Gender and Welfare State Restructuring*, edited by S. Michel and R. Mahon, 219–38. New York: Routlegde.

———. 2004. 'The Making of Local Child Daycare Regimes: Past and Future'. *Policy & Politics* 32 (1): 3–20.

Ridge, Tess. 2013. '"We Are All in This Together"? The Hidden Costs of Poverty, Recession and Austerity Policies on Britain's Poorest Children'. *Children & Society* 27 (5): 406–17. https://doi.org/10.1111/chso.12055.

Rose, Nikolas. 1996. 'Governing "Advanced" Liberal Democracies'. In *Foucault and Political Reason. Liberalism, Neo-Liberalism and Rationalities of Government*, edited by Andrew Barry, Thomas Osborne, and Nikolas Rose, 37–64. London: Routledge.

Rose, Nikolas, and Filippa Lentzos. 2017. 'Making Us Resilient: Responsible Citizens for Uncertain Times'. In *Competing Responsibilities: The Ethics and Politics of Contemporary Life*, edited by Susanna Trnka and Catherine Trundle, 27–48. Durham: Duke University Press.

Sarwar, Tahira. 2002. 'Infant Feeding Practices of Pakistani Mothers in England and Pakistan'. *Journal of Human Nutrition and Dietetics* 15 (6): 419–28.

Scott, Susie. 2009. *Making Sense of Everyday Life*. Cambridge: Polity Press.

Shore, Cris. 2017. 'Audit Culture and the Politics of Responsibility: Beyond Neoliberal Responsibilization?' In *Competing Responsibilities: The Ethics and Politics of Contemporary Life*, edited by Susanna Trnka and Catherine Trundle, 96–117. Durham: Duke University Press.

Shore, Cris, and Susan Wright. 1997. 'Policy: A New Field of Anthropology'. In *Anthropology of Policy: Critical Perspectives on Governance and Power*, edited by Cris Shore and Susan Wright, 3–34. London: Routlegde.

Strathern, Marylin. 2000. 'Introduction: New Accountabilities'. In *Audit Cultures: Anthropological Studies in Accountability, Ethics and the Academy*, edited by Marylin Strathern, 1–18. London: Routledge.

Strong, Helen, and Rebecca Wells. 2020. 'Brexit-Related Food Issues in the UK Print Media: Setting the Agenda for Post-Brexit Food Policy'. *British Food Journal* 122 (7): 2187–201. https://doi.org/10.1108/BFJ-08-2019-0582.

Stuckler, David, Aaron Reeves, Rachel Loopstra, Marina Karanikolos, and Martin McKee. 2017. 'Austerity and Health: The Impact in the UK and Europe'. *European Journal of Public Health* 27 (suppl_4): 18–21. https://doi.org/10.1093/eurpub/ckx167.

Toren, Christina. 2007. 'Sunday Lunch in Fiji: Continuity and Transformation in Ideas of the Household'. *American Anthropologist* 109 (2): 285–95.

———. 2011. 'The Stuff of Imagination: What We Can Learn from Fijian Children's Ideas About Their Lives as Adults'. *Social Analysis* 55 (1): 23–47. https://doi.org/10.3167/sa.2011.550102.

———. 2012. 'Imagining the World That Warrants Our Imagination: The Revelation of Ontogeny'. *Cambridge Anthropology* 30 (1): 64–79. https://doi.org/10.3167/ca.2012.300107.

Tronto, Joan C. 1993. *Moral Boundaries: A Political Argument for an Ethic of Care*. New York: Routlegde.

———. 2013. 'Introduction: When Care Is No Longer 'at Home''. In *Caring Democracy. Markets, Equality, and Justice*. New York: New York University Press.

Uprichard, Emma. 2008. 'Children as "Being and Becomings": Children, Childhood and Temporality'. *Children & Society* 22 (4): 303–13. https://doi.org/10.1111/j.1099-0860.2007.00110.x.

Utas, Mats. 2003. *Sweet Battlefields: Youth and Teh Liberian Civil War*. Stockholm: Lindblom & Co.

Vander Schee, Carolyn. 2009. 'Fruit, Vegetables, Fatness, and Foucault: Governing Students and Their Families through School Health Policy'. *Journal of Education Policy* 24 (5): 557–74. https://doi.org/10.1080/02680930902823047.

Vanderbeck, Robert M. and Nancy Worth. 2015. 'Introduction'. In *Intergenerational Space*, edited by Robert M. Vanderbeck and Nancy Worth. New York: Routledge.

Vertovec, Steven. 2007. 'Super-Diversity and Its Implications'. *Ethnic and Racial Studies* 30 (6): 1024–54. https://doi.org/10.1080/01419870701599465.Warming, Hanne. 2005. 'Participant Observation: A Way to Learn about Children's Perspectives'. In *Beyond Listening: Children's Perspectives on Early Childhood Services*, edited by Alison Clark, Anne-Trine Kjørholt, and Peter Moss, 51–70. Bristol: The Policy Press.

Wedel, Janine R., Cris Shore, Gregory Feldman, and Stacy Lathrop. 2005. 'Toward an Anthropology of Public Policy'. *The ANNALS of the American Academy of Political and Social Science* 600 (1): 30–51.

Wessendorf, Susanne. 2014. 'The Ethos of Mixing'. In *Commonplace Diversity: Social Relations in a Super-Diverse Context* edited by Susanne Wessendorf, 102–120. London: Palgrave Macmillan.

West, Harry G. 2000. 'Girls with Guns: Narrating the Experience of War of FRELIMO's "Female Detachment"'. *Anthropological Quarterly* 73 (4): 180–94.

Wood, Hannah, and Nikki Dyson. 2015. *1000 Things To Eat*. London: Usborne Publishing.

1 Rethinking responsibility? The state in children's everyday lives

Drawing from Bacchi and Goodwin's "What's the Problem Represented to be?" (WPR) approach (2016), this chapter will unpack official discourses around childhood obesity and sugar intake specifically, by looking at four secondary sources: Public Health England's 'Sugar Reduction Strategy' (Public Health England, Targett, and Allen 2015), the Department for Education's 'Statutory Framework for the Early Years Foundation Stage' (henceforth EYFS) (Department for Education 2017), the Children's Food Trust's 'Eat Better Start Better' (henceforth EBSB) framework (Children's Food Trust 2012), and 'The HENRY[1] Approach to Preventing Childhood Obesity' (Roberts 2015).

I have chosen these examples as they represent the perspectives of the main stakeholders that shape policy and practice in the domain of children's food: public health, early childhood education and care (ECEC) policy, and the third sector (or charity). Further, the guidelines put forward in the EYFS and EBSB were followed at Ladybird Nursery and Children's Setting, shaping the practices that happened within the setting. Similarly, the 'HENRY Approach' was implemented with parents at Ladybird and in several settings across the borough where I conducted research. The 'Sugar Reduction Strategy' represents an overarching official and mainstream narrative that has informed many children's food campaigns, and links with some of the concerns about children's diets held by official actors, practitioners, and families. By looking at the domains of public health, education, and the third (or charity) sector, I also show how the Mixed Economy of Welfare (henceforth MEW) works in practice. I suggest that the 'problems' of childhood obesity and high sugar intake have broadly been identified in official discourse as caused by 'bad' parenting practices, lack of knowledge, information and/or skills, and insufficient early intervention. This is echoed in the secondary sources that I examine, but also in the ethnographic evidence I gathered.

In examining these issues, I will explore how state policy further validates notions of individual accountability on a macro-scale, and the question of what responsibility and 'responsibilisation' mean in the context of an advanced liberal democracy will be assessed. Using a Foucauldian approach to understand ECEC and children's food policy sheds light on how notions of individual accountability and parental blame have largely dominated in these discourses, and how these impacted the everyday lives of the people I worked with. This policy context,

DOI: 10.4324/9781003297642-2

I further argue, is what creates the set of circumstances which contributes to a mismatch between the universalism of policy and the particularism of caring practices (including feeding practices).

The secondary sources: brief background

This chapter begins by analysing discourses on children and obesity in four secondary sources. The EYFS is one of the requirements to be met by early years providers, as stipulated by the Childcare Act 2006, which regulates "the powers and duties of local authorities in England and Wales in relation to the provision of childcare" (Childcare Act 2006, 1). The EYFS became mandatory for all providers in England on 3 April 2017 (Department for Education 2017, 3).[2] The Office for Standards in Education, Children's Services and Skills (Ofsted), which carry out yearly inspections of early year settings, require that providers abide by the EYFS guidelines.

The EBSB framework was developed in 2012 by the U.K. charity, The Children's Food Trust. Formed in 2005 (and originally called The School Food Trust) by the Department for Education, its mission statement was "to improve children's health by transforming food in schools" (Nursery World 2017). In 2006, the Trust initially worked on setting the school food standards in primary schools, and then in secondary schools in 2007 (ibid.). In July 2017, the charity's chief executive announced the Trust's closure, due to lack of funding.

The 'Sugar Reduction Strategy' was published by Public Health England in June 2014, following a 2015 report by the U.K.'s Scientific Advisory Committee on Nutrition that comprehensively discussed "the role of carbohydrates in cardio-metabolic, colo-rectal and oral health" (Scientific Advisory Committee on Nutrition 2015, iii). The report concludes that, "the population overall consumes more than the recommended amount of sugars and less than the recommended amount of dietary fibre," and puts forward that,

> there needs to be a change in the population's diet so that people derive a greater proportion of total dietary energy from foods that are lower in free sugars and higher in dietary fibre whilst continuing to derive approximately 50% of total dietary energy from carbohydrates.
>
> (ibid., 5–6)

The 'Sugar Reduction Strategy,' whilst not specifically addressing the early years, does outline several recommendations to families and children.

Finally, HENRY is a national charity, funded by the National Lottery and established in 2007. Its mission is to provide a preventative approach to address the risks of childhood obesity and is "commissioned by health departments as a child obesity intervention focused on children aged 0–5 years and their families" (Roberts 2015, 87–88). Whilst the intervention is open to all, it was designed with the intention of engaging families living in communities with high levels of social deprivation (ibid., 91).

Framing 'the problem' in an advanced liberal democracy

Rose contends (following Foucault) that advanced liberal democracies are defined by three characteristics: "A new relation between politics and expertise," "A new pluralization of 'social' technologies," and "A new specification of the subject of government" (1996, 54–57). In broad terms, Rose proposed that these defining features of advanced liberalism enable the act of government to become detached from the state, and the state from individuals; this is aided by the emergence of new techniques and mechanisms that enable states to govern people 'at a distance' (ibid., 57). Similarly, Lemke argues that it is governments that decide what problems are and how they should be addressed, thus also being in control of deciding what mechanisms should be used to address problems (2001, 191). He highlights, furthermore, that Foucault saw governmental practices and power relations as instrumental to the production of individuals' subjectivities (ibid.) – shaping citizens' understandings of themselves and the lives around them.

The vision of government performed 'at a distance' and as a 'producer' of citizens is the starting point of Bacchi and Goodwin's "What's the Problem Represented to be?" (henceforth WPR) approach (2016). The WPR approach problematises the assumption that policies are rational and neutral mechanisms. We are invited to think of 'problems' that policy seeks to address as *produced* by policy itself, and as such, solutions need to be similarly produced by policy through interventions that respond to specific framings of these 'problems' (Bacchi and Goodwin 2016, 16). Thus, the authors call for us to pay attention to how the explanations given for any given policy 'problem' impact people's lives, and to question the solutions presented as responding to that 'problem' (ibid.).

Their analysis is guided by six key questions:

1 What's the problem [...] represented to be in a specific policy or policies?
2 What deep-seated presuppositions or assumptions underlie this representation of the 'problem' (*problem representation*)?
3 How has this representation of the 'problem' come about?
4 What is left unproblematic in this problem representation? [...] Can the "problem" be conceptualised differently?
5 What effects (discursive, subjectification, lived) are produced by this representation of the 'problem'?
6 How and where has this representation of the "problem" been produced, disseminated and defended? How has it been and/or how can it be disrupted and replaced? (ibid., 20, original emphasis).

I will use these overarching questions to unpack how the 'problems' of childhood obesity and high sugar intake are framed in Public Health England's 'Sugar Reduction Strategy' (Public Health England, Targett, and Allen 2015), the Department for Education's EYFS (Department for Education 2017), the Children's Food Trust EBSB voluntary food and drink guidelines (Children's Food Trust 2012), and 'The HENRY Approach to Preventing Childhood Obesity' (Roberts 2015). I have chosen these examples as they illustrate the public health, ECEC policy, and third sector (or charity) perspectives, and are representative of the dominant trends and narratives about children's food and eating in the U.K. Furthermore, these guidelines were followed within Ladybird Nursery, and largely shaped the feeding practices of staff members within the setting, how children experienced their mealtimes, as well as the family interventions that I observed.[3]

Several scholars have already critiqued the ideas (often found in policy) that 'bad' parenting practices and lack of knowledge, information, and cooking skills are the issues which need to be addressed in order to solve any 'problems' related to children's eating (e.g. Murphy 2000; Caraher and Dowler 2007; Faircloth 2013; Elliott and Hore 2016; O'Connell and Brannen 2016). The U.K. policy context, which has historically framed parents, particularly working-class parents, as unqualified (e.g. Clarke 2006; Camps and Long 2012; Dermott and Pomati 2016; Sayer 2017; Lambert 2019), seems to not consider certain factors that have an impact on children's eating (such as poverty and a highly industrialised food system) in these explanations of the 'problems.' Importantly, the notions of responsibility and individual accountability have repeatedly emerged as the solutions to improve children's (and adults') eating. This, in turn, has also led official actors to put particular emphasis on early intervention as another (preventive) solution to the 'problems' of childhood obesity and high sugar intake. Before looking at the secondary sources I have chosen, a brief discussion about the definition of 'responsibility' in advanced liberal contexts will be provided.

Responsibility as a technique of government

In liberal democracies, 'choice' is "the very act that turns a person into a subject" or citizen (Mol 2008, x). This is an important consideration if choice and responsibility are understood as the processes through which individuals are governed, but also govern themselves (Lemke 2001, 91). Shore contends that the idea of responsibility is an inescapable and defining quality of contemporary society (2017, 97). Shore views responsibility as a kind of 'double-edged sword'; as an established (and internalised) normative concept, it is difficult to challenge, or to separate it from how people come to understand themselves as subjects and citizens (ibid., 100).

The assumption that society is populated by self-governing individuals is both a characteristic of, and is characterised by, advanced liberalism: it is what enables the act of government to be performed 'at a distance' (Rose 1996). This assumption also makes it easy to disregard that individuals' myriad life circumstances are what determine their 'choices' (Vander Schee 2009, 560). Much of the policy narrative that I will analyse in this chapter is underpinned by the vision that individuals are self-governing or self-regulating. This idea, by extension, was present in many of the conversations that I had with Ladybird staff and parents during my fieldwork. In many adults' feeding practices, an intention to encourage this sense of autonomy in children – epitomised in the ability to make 'healthy choices' – was also common.

Similarly, Rose and Lentzos (2017) focus on the central role that responsibility plays in modern understandings of citizenship. Taking from Elias' work on the "civilizing process" (1994), they contend that, "the practices for civilizing human subjects by turning them into responsible citizens" (2017, 28) can be understood as "citizenship projects," whereby individuals are classified as 'successful' or 'unsuccessful' citizens based on their ability to exert responsibility to varying degrees (ibid.). Whilst the question of defining children's citizenship remains a contested topic (e.g. Lister 2008; Tisdall and Punch 2012), Rose's definition of citizens as individuals "with rights to social protection and social education in return for duties of social obligation and social responsibility" (1996, 49) seemed to feature prominently in the discussions I had with staff at Ladybird and parents, and in the official discourses that informed many of their practices. In advanced liberalism, public life – the ways in which individuals relate to themselves, others, and the state – is guided by these ideals of citizenship, responsibility, and choice (Caldeira 2013, 232; Trnka and Trundle 2014, 138).

Notions of responsibility and accountability are also deeply interlinked to the 'audit culture' prevalent in the British welfare state (Trnka and Trundle 2014, 139; Shore 2017). Shore sees a clear link between ideas of responsibility and the emergence of audit and bureaucratic practices to measure accountability (2017, 98), in that institutions and individuals' actions in an advanced liberal paradigm tend to be organised around aims of efficiency, measurable outcomes, and self-surveillance (ibid., 105). This is, of course, not a linear, neat, or uncontested process, as other scholars have also noted (Mol 2008; Trnka and Trundle 2014). Yet, despite mounting evidence that the messiness and unpredictability of everyday life does not suit the 'rational' and systematic model offered to us in advanced liberalism and by policy, these overarching assumptions continue to lie at the centre of official narratives about 'healthy eating.'

The 'problems': childhood obesity and high sugar intake

Children's nutrition, particularly childhood obesity, has received increased attention from public health and government actors in recent decades (e.g. Hilton, Patterson, and Teyhan 2012; Goisis, Sacker, and Kelly 2016; Perkins and DeSousa 2018; Goisis, Martinson, and Sigle 2019). The Health & Social Care Information Centre (HSCIC) has conducted the National Child Measurement Programme (NCMP) since 2005, which entails the collection of Body Mass Index (BMI) data for children in reception (4–5 years old) and year 6 (10–11 years old) in state-maintained schools in England. Results from the NCMP report for the 2021/2022 school year show that, in reception, 10.1% of children[4] were either living with overweight or obesity (National Statistics 2022), and children in socioeconomically deprived areas were more than twice as likely to be living with overweight or obesity (ibid.). Similar trends have been recorded by the Centre for Longitudinal Studies at University College London (UCL), where results from the Millennium Cohort Study (MCS) consistently show that there is a high obesity prevalence among those born at the turn of the century (Centre for Longitudinal Studies 2014; Fitzsimons and Bann 2020).

As such, the topic of childhood obesity features predominantly in the policy documents I chose to examine between 2015 and 2019.[5] In Public Health England's

'Sugar Reduction Strategy,' obesity is mentioned in the first paragraph of the executive summary, referring to the financial burden obesity poses on the U.K.'s National Health Service (NHS):

> Consuming too many foods and drinks high in sugar can lead to weight gain and related health problems, as well as tooth decay. Almost 25% of adults, 10% of 4 to 5 year olds and 19% of 10 to 11 year olds in England are obese, with significant numbers also being overweight. Treating obesity and its consequences alone currently costs the NHS £5.1bn every year.
>
> (Public Health England 2015, 5)

Reference to childhood obesity is made once in relation to another one of Public Health England's campaigns, Change4Life:

> A key commitment PHE made last year was to encourage reduction in sugar intakes through its childhood obesity prevention campaign Change4Life (C4L). Health marketing is important as both a motivator and enabler for consumers to change their own and their families' diets and can help underpin action by others such as the food industry. It is also a key part of systems leadership work on obesity.
>
> (ibid., 34)

Indeed, information about Change4Life featured in many of the interventions I observed during fieldwork, and was a very visible campaign in the context of the early years. Change4Life posters hung in the main hallway at Ladybird, and some parents received Change4Life information pamphlets and leaflets from the staff, or during community cooking classes. The dietician that held a fortnightly clinic at Ladybird also relied on this campaign in her encounters with parents, using it to signpost them to further guidance or as support to the advice she was giving them, for example.

By a similar token, the 'HENRY Approach' points to statistics around childhood obesity (2015, 87), related health risks and financial burden on the NHS (ibid., 92), the "obesogenic environment" (ibid., 87, 91), and highlights the higher rates of childhood obesity among socioeconomically disadvantaged groups (ibid., 88, 91). Importantly, particular emphasis is placed on the early years as a time in which to intervene to prevent obesity:

> Rapid weight and obesity in the early months of life are linked to the development of long-term obesity [...] Once established, obesity is extremely difficult to reverse, and treatment of obesity in childhood and adolescence is very often unsuccessful [...] The good news is that it is easier to prevent or reverse obesity early in life, when parents are most receptive to help and support, and when children are forming enduring food preferences and eating and activity habits.
>
> (ibid., 87)

The importance of early intervention is echoed in the EBSB guidelines. In the foreword, the chief executive of Children's Food Trust states that, "with almost a quarter of children overweight or obese by the time they reach even their reception year, it's clear that supporting healthy eating can never begin too early" (Children's Food Trust 2012, 4). Statistics about children's eating and weight are introduced early in the document, alongside a list of foods that lead to overweight and obesity in children (foods high in fat, sugar, and salt) (ibid., 7). Given that this framework was put together and published to encourage early years settings to develop and implement their own 'food policy,' its main focus is to "[help] children maintain a healthy weight as they grow" (ibid., 55). The guidelines provide detailed information about food groups, menu plans, portion sizes, and initiatives to involve both parents and children in this campaign. Childcare settings, such as Ladybird, that followed the EBSB framework needed to create and maintain a 'portfolio' with evidence showing how their food policy was being implemented, and staff members involved in feeding children regularly had to attend training sessions to update their knowledge and practice. EBSB is also directly linked to the EYFS:

> This guide has been developed to help early years providers and practitioners to meet the Early Years Foundation Stage (EYFS) welfare requirement for the provision of healthy, balanced and nutritious food and drink [...] Involving parents and their children in food and drink provision is an important aspect of the Early Years Foundation Stage framework.
>
> (ibid., 6)

The campaign was thus heavily audited in all the settings that implemented it, and the local educational authority did this by creating a 'staged' assessment system, in which childcare settings enrolled in the campaign needed to fulfil three requirements. First, early years staff need to be trained to have "increased food, nutrition and healthy cooking knowledge, skills and confidence" (Mucavele et al. 2014, 67). Following this training, childcare settings needed to "[improve] healthier food provision for children aged one to five" (ibid., 68). The final outcome for settings to reach a 'Stage 3' assessment by the local authority was to evidence, "Increased food and nutrition knowledge and practical cooking skills for parents and families" (ibid.). In the words of Diana, the programme lead for the EBSB programme in the borough where I conducted fieldwork:

> *By achieving a Stage 3, that's when we're really confident that the menu quality is good, that the setting has got the knowledge and skills to be able to plan nutritionally balanced menus. And also when they get to Stage 3 we're confident that they have...that healthy eating is threaded through everything that they do. So it's like a whole setting approach and it is threaded through all of their curriculum. And when we get to that point we know that the setting can maintain that quality – semi-structured interview, July 2017.*

This holistic vision advocated by the EBSB approach exemplifies how public health, education, and family intervention policies intertwine in official discourses about children's food and eating.

A sense of urgency is laced through these documents: appealing to the financial burden obesity poses on the NHS adds to this rhetoric, as well as the 'irreversibility' of being classified as obese from an early age. Several scholars have called the 'crisis' narrative of childhood obesity into question (see, e.g. Warin et al. 2008; Maher, Fraser, and Lindsay 2010; Moffat 2010), and measures such as the BMI are also increasingly deemed problematic by social scientists and health professionals alike (Kelly and Daniels 2017). Yet, whilst the official narratives around these issues (particularly the underlying assumptions about causality, the irreversibility of habits learnt at an early age, and the interaction between moralised notions of 'acceptable bodies' and biomedicine) should be questioned and examined, the risks and adverse health outcomes related to obesity should not be ignored, particularly the role these play in widening health inequalities in the U.K. (Rougeaux et al. 2017; Schrecker 2017; Pearce et al. 2019). Indeed, as Brewis contends, "obesity can be framed as a social and political – as much as a medical – issue" (2011, 2; Rees et al. 2011; see also Yates-Doerr 2015).

Parallel to the issue of childhood obesity, the matter of children's high sugar intake has gained equal prominence in official and mainstream discourse, around the world (e.g. Evans et al. 2011) and in the U.K. (Albon 2005; Gibson et al. 2016; Evans 2017). As shown in the policy documents above, the consumption of sugary drinks and foods has been framed as a cause for concern because of its association with childhood obesity. Nonetheless, I am treating it and discussing this as a separate 'problem' in this chapter because of its links to other health issues, such as tooth decay, as well as onset of type-2 diabetes and cardiovascular diseases later in life (Gibson et al. 2016). The U.K.'s Scientific Advisory Committee on Nutrition advises that, "the population average of free sugars[6] should not exceed 5% of total dietary energy" (Scientific Advisory Committee on Nutrition 2015, 183). Similarly to obesity, sugar consumption is also a highly moralised theme in discussions about children's feeding practices. As I will show in subsequent chapters, parents struggled between the intention to limit their children's sugar intake and the desire to also satisfy their children's preference for certain treats – indeed, expressing love and care through food can also entail acts of nutritional transgression. The contradictory cultural paradigm which suggests that sweet foods are foods for children (whilst sugar is simultaneously demonised) also plays a significant role in shaping the relation between food, care, and sociality (Albon 2015; Hansen and Kristensen 2017).

What are the factors that are assumed to make the 'problems' persist?

In the U.K., three broad explanations for any 'problems' associated to children's eating have predominated in official and mainstream discourse: inadequate parenting practices, lack of knowledge and/or skills, and insufficient early intervention. These are greatly interlinked, and many of the initiatives I observed during fieldwork tried to address the three in conjunction. This was particularly so in the case of HENRY. Being specifically aimed at the early years, the charity responds to long-lasting (and periodically renewed) policy emphasis on early intervention in England (and the U.K. at large), and also places specific focus on parenting practices:

> HENRY aims to foster loving parenting styles that nonetheless hold firm boundaries with regard to eating and behaviour. Evidence shows that parenting efficacy is a key risk factor for child obesity.
>
> (Roberts 2015, 89)

'Knowledge' and 'skills' also appear on HENRY's policy framework, aiming to improve these among the early years workforce, and parents by extension:

> HENRY 2-day training courses equip practitioners with the skills, knowledge and confidence to help parents adopt a healthy family lifestyle right from the start, and to respond effectively to signs of rapid weight gain in infants and young children.
>
> (ibid., 90)

Similarly, the EBSB guidelines emphasise that communication (i.e. providing information) between childcare settings and families is fundamental to encourage parents and children to make 'healthy choices,' suggesting that behaviour change should be one of the outcomes sought when designing and implementing their own EBSB food policy: "Your [the setting's] approach to food offers an opportunity to encourage children and their families to eat well and to provide information and healthy food choices [sic]" (Children's Food Trust 2012, 45). One way to do this, the framework suggests, is to "provide information for parents and carers on the routine for meals and snacks in your setting, to help them plan their child's routine at home" (ibid.). The link between the early years setting and home environment is clear in these documents, 'responsibilising' childcare workers and, through them, parents.

Providing better access to information across the population is also cited in the 'Sugar Reduction Strategy' as one of the recommendations to address the 'problem' of high sugar intake (Public Health England 2015, 8). Increased consumer knowledge, furthermore, is described as particularly relevant in the case of parents:

> Challenges remain around the adoption of the portion size recommendation for fruit juice. Large cartons generally make it difficult to know the size of a portion without measuring it and small cartons (aimed at the lunchbox market) predominantly contain more than the 150ml (generally around 200ml). *There is an opportunity for industry to make it easier for parents to give their children just the recommended 150ml portion* whether this is by marking portion sizes on the side of cartons or other uses of labelling to highlight this; or by reducing the size of small cartons to correspond with the recommended portion size.
>
> (ibid., 36, original emphasis)

Both the 'HENRY Approach' and the 'Sugar Reduction Strategy' mention the food environment and industry as factors that contribute to obesity and high sugar intake. The 'Sugar Reduction Strategy,' in particular, proposes market-related solutions to high sugar intake as its first two recommendations in its executive summary (ibid., 7). Nonetheless, it is worth mentioning that the matter of corporate or industry accountability is still very much tied to notions of individual responsibility. The implications of this will be further discussed in the next chapter.

Childhood obesity and sugar intake are not specifically mentioned in the EYFS; nonetheless, its link with the EBSB campaign has already been noted. Further, the themes of widening access to knowledge and information to improve food standards in early years settings (Department for Education 2017, 21–22, 28), and of creating synergy between early years practitioners and parents (ibid., 5–7, 32–33) are also salient. Food in the early years context can thus be regarded as a 'pedagogical tool.'[7]

Teaching children about 'healthy choices' and table manners featured highly on the list of priorities of some staff who worked at Ladybird. In this narrative, the link between eating habits and the 'civilised body' – "the body that is tightly contained, consciously managed, subject to continual self-surveillance as well as surveillance on the part of others" (Lupton 1996, 22) – is salient. As Lupton contends, there are numerous expectations and values related to food and eating that have been shaped by the idea of the 'civilised body.' This is an important point to keep in mind when questioning official concerns and responses related to children's eating. For example, concern for children's health can often also be entangled with an aversion towards fatness, which in the U.K. continues to be associated with a whole range of negative social categories (Evans et al. 2011, 335). It is therefore important to acknowledge that just as the biomedical sphere informs social practices, so can social norms and moral understandings of food and bodies influence biomedical discourses (Evans, Rich, and Davies 2004, 382).

Implicit in the guidelines I have discussed are the assumptions that: increased knowledge will lead to behaviour change; that the early years are a crucial time for intervention because, "Children develop quickly in the early years and a child's experiences between birth and age five have a major impact on their future life chances" (Department of Education 2017, 5); and that "parenting, emotional well-being and whole-family lifestyle [is] a foundation for enabling young children to develop healthy food preferences" (Roberts 2015, 88). Failure to address these areas, therefore, is assumed to make the problems persist. These domains continue to receive attention from a diversity of sectors in the MEW, with both state and private actors working together to achieve similar goals, but through often different or contradictory means.

It needs to be noted, nonetheless, that whilst these three factors (inadequate parenting practices, lack of information/knowledge, and insufficient early intervention) have been given prominence in official discourse in recent decades, there has also been a contemporary move towards acknowledging the influence of the food environment and industry on children and their families. As shown above, this is particularly so in the case of the 'Sugar Reduction Strategy,' and its recommendations have been widely adopted in several 'healthy eating' campaigns, such as Change4Life. This strategy has also called for there to be better regulations around price promotions in the retail and catering sectors; to limit marketing of high sugar foods and drinks (particularly to children); to impose a 'sugar tax' or 'levy' on high sugar foods and drinks; as well as to improve, regulate, and monitor the standards of food provided in public sector institutions, such as schools and hospitals (Public Health England 2015, 7–8). The benefits and drawbacks of these proposals are also subject to debate, which is beyond the scope of this book. Yet, whilst this shift in emphasis from the individual to the 'environmental' factors impacting people's diets is certainly a welcome change, this too should be treated with caution, particularly if issues of access to food and health inequalities are to be properly accounted for (e.g. Ingram et al. 2013; Throsby 2018). In particular, the notion that everyone is willing and able to make the same choices when presented with the same options in the free-market economy needs to be evaluated (Mol 2008, 74–78; O'Connell and Brannen 2016, 3); this will also be discussed in Chapter 2.

What is the historical context underlying the assumptions made in official discourse?

Emphasis on individual accountability in policy discourse emerged in the early 1980s, first during the Thatcher years, and has continued under subsequent Conservative and New Labour administrations. As Sayer argues, within this vision of a 'meritocratic' society there has been little regard for the impact that wider economic processes have on people's ability to make 'choices,' with individuals being held almost entirely responsible for their life outcomes (2017, 157). This paradigm has had direct consequences on family intervention and public health policies in the U.K. In particular, it has made public health discourse increasingly individualised, and this contributes to reinforcing perceptions about parental blame in discussions about children's feeding practices. Alongside this rhetoric of individual accountability, a narrative of economic profitability and return on investments has also permeated the policy discourses I am examining here, which other scholars have also pointed out (e.g. Moss and Petrie 2000; Penn 2007; Lee and Motzkau 2011).

Importantly, appealing to the notion of 'human capital' has significant implications in how citizenship is construed in these policy narratives. As Macvarish has discussed for the New Labour years, during which policy efforts to 'support families' were put in place, family interventions to redress parental behaviour that was perceived as deficient became central as a way to address the 'problem' of 'social exclusion' (rather than tackling the causes of inequality) (2014, 83–84).

As well as being pervasive in family intervention policies, public health discourse has also become imbued with appeals to improve 'health behaviours' to safeguard the economic integrity of state institutions. This is shown, for example, in the framing of childhood obesity as a financial burden to the NHS in the 'Sugar Reduction Strategy' (Public Health England 2015, 5, 9, 14–15) and the 'HENRY Approach' (Roberts 2015, 92) – and this also has implications for how citizenship and individual responsibility are construed. As Petersen and Lupton argue, 'good health' signifies 'virtuous citizenship' in advanced liberalism, as it guarantees continued productivity over the better part of people's lifetime (1996, 67).

Alongside these claims to economic efficiency – and, arguably, because of them – a culture of audit and assessment (Power 1999) has established itself within this policy context, which Shore contends has created a transformation in how "the management of human relations" (2017, 104) and self-surveillance are enacted. Shore argues that "with its hallmark emphasis on scrutiny, inspection, surveillance, cost accounting, and compliance, audit has become a powerful technology for producing responsible subjects" (ibid., 104–5). Furthermore, this form of 'measurable accountability' adds to the semblance of rationality and neutrality of institutions, organisations, and bureaucracies (ibid., 106). Indeed, the U.K.'s MEW model is very much based around these premises, and measurability and accountability become particularly central when different providers are positioned as competitors that offer similar welfare services (Alcock and Scott 2014, 101).

The rhetoric of audit and assessment is laced through the 'Sugar Reduction Strategy,' the EYFS, the EBSB framework, and the 'HENRY Approach.' Audit is fundamental across institutions, and particularly so for the survival of the voluntary and charity sectors. Service providers in this domain need to provide evidence of measurable outcomes to continue receiving state and private funds to finance their activities. As such, the last pages of the HENRY guidelines are devoted to providing statistical data showing the 'impact' that the intervention has had since its inception (Roberts 2015, 91–92). This section of the document is also framed in the 'return on investments' language of audit culture:

> The positive impact of HENRY's holistic approach on family lifestyle, as well as children's food consumption and activity levels, suggests that prevention in the early years can make a real difference. Demonstrating return on investment in prevention is notoriously difficult, and we welcome the opportunity of the National Institute for Health Research-funded trial to further national and international understanding of the long-term impact of investment at the start of life.
>
> (ibid., 92)[8]

These are thus the historical and political conditions that underlie the representation of childhood obesity and high sugar intake in official discourse. Whilst recently there has been increased acknowledgement of the 'environmental' factors that cause these 'problems' to arise, it is also evident that an emphasis on individual accountability and audit culture still tend to dominate in these discussions (Ulijaszek and McLennan 2016, 407). By maintaining this focus, other factors that contribute to these 'problems' can in turn be overlooked.

What is ignored in official framings of the 'problems'?

Notions of individual accountability have permeated family intervention and public health discourses in Britain. However, an area that has not been sufficiently addressed by policymakers and public health officials are the structural factors that affect people's food habits.

As discussed above, tighter food industry regulations have been proposed by Public Health England in their 'Sugar Reduction Strategy' (Public Health England 2015, 7–8), showing a potential turn in how the 'problem' of high sugar intake will be framed within official discourse. Nonetheless, when looking specifically at policies directed at families and children, what features prominently are notions of parental accountability and equipping children with the 'right' knowledge to make 'healthy choices,' whilst the food environment and industry are almost absent. For example, "[increasing] parenting efficacy" (Roberts 2015, 89) is a central aim of the 'HENRY Approach.' The issue of the food environment is mentioned twice in this framework, in which the need for an "attitude change" (ibid., 87) and "building resilience" (ibid., 91) towards the U.K.'s 'obesogenic environment' is cited. The EYFS also alludes, in vague terms, to moralised ideals about parenting practices, stating in its Introduction that, "*Good parenting* and high quality early learning together provide the foundation children need to make the most of their abilities and talents as they grow up" (Department for Education 2017, 5, own emphasis). The notion that early years workers and parents should communicate and 'work together' to improve children's eating is thus present in these guidelines, and by extension in the EBSB framework, which seeks to help settings meet the welfare requirements laid out in the EYFS. Parents also feature (briefly) in the 'Sugar Reduction Strategy,' where improved labelling on food products is suggested to help parents make better informed purchases for their children (Public Health England 2015, 36). Teaching parents how to adequately read labels is also central in the Change4Life campaign (which relies greatly on the recommendations developed in the 'Sugar Reduction Strategy').

By emphasising parents' position in determining their children's diets, the other social relations children engage in (with other adults and peers alike) are underemphasised. In fact, the various contexts children eat in, and the other people they eat with, play a significant role. Qvortrup (2005) has pointed out that a defining feature of 'modern childhood' is a view of children as marginal in the public sphere, as they are predominantly perceived as relating to their family units and educational institutions, rather than all adults and society in general (2005, 4). This is the view of childhood that continues to predominate in English policymaking. In the context of food and eating, this reinforces the normative assumption that parents shape their children's eating in a unidirectional and authoritative way (Curtis, Stapleton, and James 2011, 435).

When adhering to a more traditional view of the family unit, the matter of gender can also be ignored in official discourse of children's food and eating. This is clear, for example, in the 'HENRY Approach'; by using the neutral term 'parents' the question of who engages with this intervention and who is in charge of foodwork (still predominantly mothers) is obscured. By not adequately addressing the issue of gender, the question of 'choice' is also not properly represented. In the words of Sally, one of the early years practitioners that I met early on in my fieldwork:

Something I have learnt from my work is about all the different family units. Money and culture in the family unit are all linked to food. Because if the mother is cooking but the money is coming from the father, the mother doesn't have much choice in what she cooks for her children, she's limited. They are all linked, everything, money, culture, education, it's hard to separate one thing and not see that everything is connected – semi-structured interview, November 2016.

Taking for granted that it is women that carry out most of the foodwork is not only detrimental to mothers who are out of employment, but also to working mothers, who continue to be framed as those to be blamed for children's 'bad' diets, both in official and mainstream discourse (O'Connell and Brannen 2016, 13). The link between maternal employment and childhood obesity had gained attention again in 2019, after the publication of a study drawing from the U.K. Millennium Cohort Study, in which data shows that "maternal employment during childhood increases children's BMI" (Fitzsimons and Pongiglione 2019, 8). The research caused wide media controversy, with headlines such as "Nice work, Mum: you've turned me into a lazy lardy" (*Times* 2019) appearing on one of Britain's leading newspapers. Emphasis on parental accountability diverts attention from the structural and cultural factors that frame some parents as 'inefficient' by policymakers.

Finally, whilst the secondary sources I have discussed in this chapter all refer to the vulnerability of lower income families, the emphasis on behaviour change shifts focus away from the issue of access to adequate resources (not only food, but also appropriate housing or fuel). For example, the kind of food budgets families have available to them are not referred to anywhere in the 'HENRY Approach,' even though this is a charity that specifically works with families living in areas of high deprivation (Roberts 2015, 91). This is surprising, given that balancing a family budget in the wake of rising food prices is increasingly a challenge for many parents in England, not only for those at the bottom of the income distribution, as most children growing up in poverty have at least one parent in paid work (O'Connell and Brannen 2016, 44–50; O'Connell et al. 2018). Stating that children and families at the lower end of the socio-economic spectrum are at higher risk of being obese or consume more sugary foods, without adequately accounting for the material constraints that might lead to this, seems contradictory.[9]

However, it is not only the material and time constraints of families that tend to be overlooked in official discourse, but also those of the early years settings to which these initiatives are promoted. This was a recurring issue during the time I spent at Ladybird. For example, whilst rolling out the EBSB campaign, the local council had simultaneously stopped providing funding to provide fruit as snacks in state-maintained settings, so Ladybird depended on families' donations of fruit to the school. The limited amount of staff (not only at Ladybird but several other settings in the borough) meant that often not all the staff were able to go to the EBSB training sessions. In some cases (including at Ladybird) settings did not have kitchen facilities to prepare food on site, not enough time, or not enough qualified staff to prepare food. Nonetheless, having enough funding to meet the voluntary standards was the main barrier that many early years settings were facing.

Indeed, the issue of the cost of food was mentioned several times as a barrier during an EBSB course that I attended with Joyce and Kate, two of Ladybird's early years practitioners. One of the activities we were asked to do during the session was to write a weekly menu plan drawing from the EBSB nutrition and portion guidelines. In my fieldnotes from that day I wrote:

> *Rachel [the nutritionist leading the session] asks for volunteers to come forward to suggest a menu for their morning and afternoon sessions each day of the week. She says that in the menus there needs to be a balance and variety of foods coming from each food group [following the 'Eatwell Guide' – Figure 1.1], and that, "balance and variety is the key to healthy eating." After we are done, the nutritionist shows us a sample menu from the EBSB handbook we were given at the beginning of the session; Rachel asks the group, "Looking at this menu, what do you think?" and one of the participants says, "Costly!" This reminds me of a comment that Joyce made to me at another session we attended, where she told me that these courses "never address the costs of providing healthy food" – fieldnotes, March 2017.*

The matter of not being able to meet the 'healthy food' standards promoted to early years workers was echoed by Robert, the extended services manager[10] at Ladybird who was also involved in designing the EBSB 'food policy' for the setting. In a semi-structured interview, he told me:

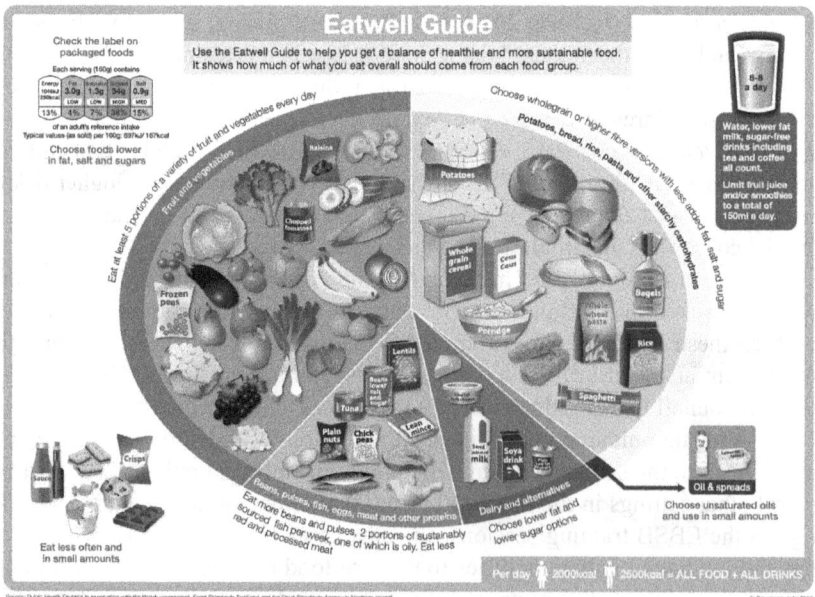

Figure 1.1 The Eatwell Guide. 2016. Public Health England in association with the Welsh Government, Food Standards Scotland and the Food Standards Agency in Northern Ireland. Available from: https://www.nhs.uk/Livewell/Goodfood/Documents/The-Eatwell-Guide-2016.pdf.

What we're able to charge parents doesn't meet anywhere near the cost of running it [tea-club], and there's no support from the local authority in running an extended day service. So thinking about what do you provide, and with really no budget, is tough – semi-structured interview, August 2018.

Thus, similarly to the issues mentioned above in relation to the 'HENRY Approach,' not adequately assessing the budget available to settings in which EBSB was being rolled out poses some problems. In our interview, Diana (the EBSB programme lead for the borough) mentioned this was one of the goals of promoting the initiative within the borough:

What we wanted to do was to target the early years providers that had higher numbers of children from poor socioeconomic backgrounds. So that's like the free school meal equivalent for early years, which is the children that would meet the criteria for the free, funded, two-year olds [places at nursery]. So we were trying to target the settings that were taking those funded two year old children because we felt that by intervening early, i.e. at two as opposed to four, then hopefully we would be able to change some of the habits and change the diet in the hope that that would influence their outcome later on. So one of our main target groups were settings with funded two year olds, and we wanted to engage as many as them as possible on the programme, and we wanted to change as many as them as possible to the Stage 3 outcome – semi-structured interview, July 2017.

Within a rationale guided by audit culture and the need to produce measurable outcomes (e.g. encouraging settings to achieve a 'Stage 3' assessment), the material constraints of both the settings, and the families to whom certain interventions are promoted, seem to be overlooked.

What impact do these official discourses have on people's daily lives?

A prevailing argument in available scholarship on 'responsibility' and 'choice' suggests that these notions have had a significant impact on peoples' subjectivities in Euro-American contexts (e.g. Lemke 2001; Mol 2008; Vander Schee 2009). Whilst I do not think I can make claims about participants' subjectivities, it is certainly the case that many of the practices and ideas that staff and parents shared with me in the time we spent together mirrored the official rhetoric I have explored in this chapter. Exploring what it meant for participants to abide by these guidelines revealed the various contradictions that emerge when official discourses become embedded in people's daily lives.

In the case of staff at Ladybird, the matter of sugar avoidance became an even more contested issue in January 2017, when new voluntary food guidelines for early years settings were introduced and it was suggested that children's fruit consumption should be restricted to avoid high sugar intakes. This caused some confusion among staff, as I noted in my fieldnotes:

It is 3 p.m.: almost time for teaclub. Ruby, who is running the session today, is setting up the table, while Joyce [the lead early years practitioner] and I are preparing the children's snacks. Ruby asks Joyce if she can include vegetables on the children's snack plates; after searching in the fridge, Joyce says that we don't have any vegetables. Since the centre relies on families' donations to provide fresh food as snacks, Ruby says she thinks we need to start asking parents to specifically donate vegetables, alongside fruit. This is because during a training course she has recently attended she was told that, "A plate of fruit is like a plate of sugar," and attendees were thus advised to reduce the amount of fruit that children consume during the day. Having worked in a few different state schools for over fifteen years, mostly in food-related roles, Ruby admits that she found this recommendation surprising. She tells me, "Every so often they come up with something that needs to be changed. I never thought it would be fruit" – fieldnotes, January 2017.

Indeed, fresh fruit is generally portrayed as a 'healthy food' in public health messages such as the 'Eatwell Guide' (Figure 1.1), and it was commonly held knowledge among both staff and parents that this is a 'good' snack to give children. Yet, the exchange between Ruby and Joyce during tea-club speaks quite strongly of the fluid and contradictory meanings that food can acquire in everyday life, largely as a result of an increased reliance of numerical representations of dietary information (Caldwell 2014, 67). Official discourse, in this case, is opposed to 'common sense' knowledge about what might be 'good' food for children. As illustrated in the above vignette, fruit, normally highly valued, can also become a source of dreaded sugar. The medicalisation and 'numerisation' of children's food has contributed to downplaying experiential and embodied knowledge (Lupton 1996) of food and eating, through an overemphasis on portion sizes and nutritional values (Fischler 2011; Caldwell 2014). This created anxiety both among childcare practitioners and parents, as often came across quite poignantly during my observations at the fortnightly dietician's clinic at Ladybird:

During a consultation that I shadowed at the dietician's clinic, Kevin's mother, Yang, reported that he had started to eat finger-sized pieces of vegetables, cheese, and noodles. She asked Freya [the dietician] for confirmation of how big the cheese portions should be. Freya indicated it should be half of her thumb. Yang then asked, "But isn't cheese too salty for him?" to which Freya responded by saying that we should indeed be careful not to give too much salt to infants. Freya recommended that she should not give Kevin cheese more than once a day.
[A few weeks later]
I caught up with Yang during a stay and play session at the children's centre today, and I asked her how Kevin's eating had been since we last saw each other at the dietician's clinic. She told me that things were going well overall, but she also anxiously asked me if I remembered how big Freya had said a portion of cheese should be, as she still was not sure if she was "getting it right" – fieldnotes, March 2017.

Yang's confusion was warranted: the suggestion that she feed Kevin food with a high protein content (such as cheese) clashed with the advice that children should not be fed salty foods, tapping into a wider anxiety about feeding Kevin the 'right' way. Even in the highly detailed EBSB guidelines, the 'healthy' amount of any given food that children should consume was often unclear. Further, the potential for 'good food' to become 'bad' seems to always be prevalent, like in Yang's situation or the case of having to limit children's fruit intake at tea-club. 'Choice' and 'responsibility' can take on a dangerous quality in a context where dietary recommendations contradict each other.

Alongside creating such contradictions, a nutrition-driven approach to food and eating contributes to the further entrenchment of a narrative of individual accountability in public health discourse. Again, this extends into a culture of parental blame (Faircloth 2013): if parents are being given all the available information about what to feed their children, then they are to be held accountable if their children are not eating 'healthily.' The way in which the public health domain contributes to this narrative in the everyday lives of families was particularly perceptible during my observations at the dietician's clinic at Ladybird. One day, I shadowed one of Freya's (the dietician) appointments with a couple who often brought their baby to sessions at the children's centre. Their reason for going in that day was that their child often had diarrhoea. The problem persisted although he had tested negative for cow's milk protein allergy, and they wanted to hear Freya's opinion and seek for further advice on how to improve his situation. In my fieldnotes from this session I noted:

> As the visit progresses, Freya goes through some routine questions she needs to ask parents, including, "From a scale from one to ten how would you rate your child's overall health?" This seems to make the mother quite uncomfortable and she hesitates, which Freya notices. Freya says apologetically that she realises that this is a strange question, and that she "doesn't know why we have to do it." After some more hesitation and some back and forth with her partner, the baby's mother says that, excluding these occasional episodes of diarrhoea, she would rate her son's health as a '9' – fieldnotes, December 2016.

Several of the themes discussed in this chapter are at play in this vignette. As well as representing the 'numerisation' of children's health, and a rather overt form of scrutinising parents, the question of 'rating' the health of one's child speaks quite poignantly of the extent to which 'audit culture' is also embedded in the daily lives of families (Shore 2017), and how it contributes to the responsibilisation of parents. Freya's attempt to reassure the baby's parents by saying 'she doesn't know why' she has to ask them this question also mirrors the notion that official actors are often guided by arbitrary bureaucratic processes, which in turn lead to more inconsistent policy 'results' (Gupta 2012, 6). Indeed, at times it seemed that rather than placating parents' anxieties, parents' visits to Freya's clinic exacerbated their worries. As I wrote in my fieldnotes from another session I observed at the clinic:

The mother expresses her frustration that whatever she does to encourage her twin sons to eat never seems to be enough. She says, "All the [public health/social] services give you all this advice, and it's great that they exist, but then you're the one who has to go home and implement it, and you're just like... bloody hell" – fieldnotes, December 2016.

This encounter at the clinic mirrors Mol's claim that "as patient customers," faced with a range of options to choose from, "we are left alone" (2008, 16). Parents are expected to make the best 'choices' for their children, informed by policies and interventions that often do not adequately address the varied time, monetary, or other constraints that might prevent them from making these 'choices.' Yet, despite these shortcomings, perceptible to parents and many of the actors that I engaged with over the course of my fieldwork, current framings of 'problems' related to children's eating continue to hold authority in official and mainstream discourse.

How do these representations of the 'problems' continue to hold authority in the public domain?

To explore how 'better' parenting, early intervention, and increased knowledge and skills continue to be framed as the solutions to the 'problems' of childhood obesity and high sugar intake, I turn to Eisenberg's work on public policy. Eisenberg defines policy communities as 'entities with power' (2011, 102) and as "contested political spaces [in which] the questions addressed are 'Whose voices prevail?' and 'How are their discourses made authoritative?'" (ibid.). I have argued that the historical and political conditions that have predominated in British policymaking – rooted in advanced liberalism – has contributed to the entrenchment of individual accountability and audit culture in official discourse about childhood obesity and high sugar intake. I have also shown some of the tangible ways in which these discourses translated into practice in the everyday lives of practitioners and parents, leading to contradictions and anxiety, and undermining the social value of food.

A number of scholars, following Foucault, have suggested that in the context of advanced liberalism, the notion of 'expertise' is fundamental to enact governmentality (Rose 1996, 50; Shore and Wright 1997, 8–9). Within this socio-political model, authority and 'expertise' are deeply tied together. In my ethnography, there are a variety of actors positioned as 'experts' in the discourse of children's food and eating: the staff at Ladybird, the people leading HENRY sessions and community cooking courses, as well as the dietician. Certainly, there were also different levels of 'expertise' that each actor held depending on their qualifications and experiences. For example, in looking at how the EBSB programme was being rolled out, I could notice the different levels and sectors that each of these 'experts' were positioned in.

At the very top of this 'policy community' was Diana, the programme lead for the EBSB programme introduced earlier. The themes of early intervention, improved knowledge and skills, and parenting practices were salient when she explained the implementation of the programme within the borough. Notions of audit and assessment were also central during the interview I conducted with her:

FV: When did 'Eat Better Start Better' start in [the borough]?

D: It must have been...2014. So the head of early years [in the local education authority] requested that some training was provided using the EBSB national guidelines. And that came about because of [the borough's] high obesity levels at the time. Because of the high obesity levels there was an under five year olds obesity strategy group, and that was headed by early years and someone in public health. Basically they had a few different work-streams linked to the obesity reduction agenda, and one of the work-streams was around upscaling the knowledge and skills of early years practitioners working with under fives to improve food policy in early years settings.
[...]

FV: You said earlier that since EBSB began there have been very positive results, with a significant decrease in obesity levels. Can you say more about that?

D: Well, [the borough] still has got one of the highest obesity rates in the reception years. Even though the trajectory is kind of positive, in that last year there are more children of a healthy weight than there has been when we started measuring, but we still have very high obesity rates. So we think it's on the right track, but there's still a lot of work to do. But I know that, according to recent research, it's the emphasis you put before they start school that will make the biggest difference. So that's why running a programme like this is so important [...] And we've got case-study evidence that suggests that there has been a behaviour change with the parents. Also we've got evidence to suggest that sometimes by working with the children, the children then are influencing the parents' choices, with things like packed lunches.

At the level below the programme lead, I met Rachel, a paediatric nutritionist who ran the EBSB courses to train early years practitioners. In the session I attended in March 2017, which she led, she emphasised the importance of the 'Eatwell Guide' (Figure 1.1) as a model on which snack times should be based. Similarly to Diana, Rachel also mentioned the link the programme sought to make between the early years settings and the home environment. In my fieldnotes from that day, I wrote:

Rachel explains that the EBSB guidelines see all snack times in stay and play sessions as "an informal way to model what mealtimes can be like [at home]," as a way to provide parents "guidance in a non-threatening way."

Whilst Rachel repeated in the session how important early years practitioners' roles were in achieving this, several of the attendees were sceptical. As noted earlier, many of them (including Joyce and Kate) mentioned restricted budgets and a limited number of staff as impediments to achieving the standards Rachel was promoting. Nonetheless, practitioners who were trained under this scheme were positioned as the 'experts' in the level below Rachel's, and were those through whom the messages of the programme were communicated to children and parents. At Ladybird, Joyce and Kate were known to be two points of contact if parents had any concerns about their children's eating. They would then share what they had learnt in their training, refer the families to Freya, or invite them to the cooking classes occasionally offered at the centre. Meanwhile, Ruby (who ran breakfast and tea-clubs at Ladybird) was in charge of updating the portfolio to show the local education authority the progress that Ladybird was making in implementing the EBSB guidelines (a task which Rachel also talked about at length during the training session). Aside from collaborating with Robert on planning the menus, Ruby also spoke at length about healthy eating to the children, and often centred some of the afternoon activities on this theme. For example, Figure 1.2 shows a collection of some of the drawings the children made of their favourite vegetables, which Ruby photographed to include in the portfolio.

In exploring this final question (How do representations of the 'problems' continue to hold authority in the public domain?) guided by Bacchi and Goodwin's WPR approach (2016), this chapter shows on way in which specific framings of

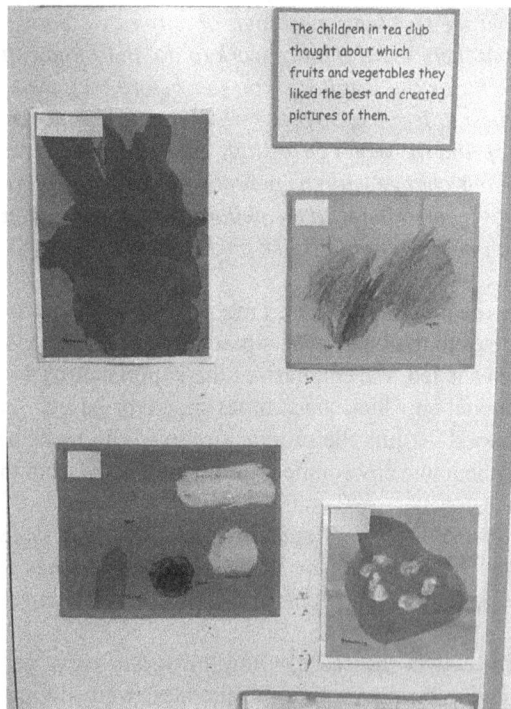

Figure 1.2 Children's drawings of their favourite vegetables.
Photograph by the author.

childhood obesity and high sugar intake as 'problems' continue to hold authority in the context in which I conducted fieldwork. There were different levels at which 'expertise' was filtered down in the 'policy community' I researched: the level of the local government, the level of public health, and the level of the early years practitioners. I have also shown that there are several policy domains that overlapped in these discussions: education, public health, and family intervention. Despite coming from different angles, all actors belonging to these three domains (both private and public) seemed to frame the 'problems' equally, and had similar approaches to 'solve' them.

Nonetheless, I say above that this is *one* of the ways in which these discourses continue to maintain authority in the public domain because reality is, of course, much more complex than this. To explore this further, in the next chapter I move on to looking at the food industry's role in upholding these official representations, and the contradictions that also arise when considering the impact of this domain in people's everyday lives.

Notes

1 HENRY is an acronym for 'Health, Exercise, Nutrition for the Really Young.'
2 The EYFS has been updated since the time fieldwork was conducted, and published in March 2021. It is still a requirement for Ofsted that all early years settings comply with EYFS guidelines.
3 Each of these domains will be explored in detail in Chapters 4, 5, and 6, respectively.
4 Of 585,750 children measured. These statistics represent an increase from the 9.5% prevalence of children in reception years living with overweight or obesity (of 610,435 children measured) in the NCMP results from the 2017/2018 school year (Stats Team, NHS Digital 2018), which were the latest available at the time when this research was conducted.
5 The 'Statutory framework for the early years foundation stage' refers to children's diets more generally, however I have also chosen to examine these guidelines for the themes of responsibility and audit it uses to outline dietary recommendations, and because it is the framework that early years settings are required to follow in order to get a positive Ofsted report. Ladybird abided by these guidelines.
6 "This comprises all monosaccharides [most basic unit of carbohydrate e.g. glucose, fructose] and disaccharides [a 'double sugar' comprised of two monosaccharides, e.g. sucrose] added to foods [...] plus sugars naturally present in honey, syrups and unsweetened fruit juices. Under this definition lactose when naturally present in milk and milk products is excluded" (Scientific Advisory Committee on Nutrition 2015, 4).
7 This concept will be explored in detail in Chapter 3.
8 The HENRY Approach has received media attention, as its implementation has been linked to a drop in childhood obesity rates in Leeds (Boseley 2019).
9 This contradiction has also been explored in the United States by Greenhalgh and Carney (2014), who assess the failures of public health campaigns that seek to raise awareness about the risks of obesity among the Latino community. These approaches, the authors argue, further exclude minorities that are already considered 'failed' citizens, instead of addressing the structural inequalities that are at the heart of the health outcomes in this community (*ibid*, 23).
10 Robert's role as extended services manager involved organising the activities families attended at the children's centre, such as cooking classes, 'stay and play' sessions,

English as a second or foreign language (ESOL) classes for parents, among other initiatives that can be regarded as an extension (or as supporting) welfare services.

References

Albon, Deborah. 2005. 'Approaches to the Study of Children, Food and Sweet Eating: A Review of the Literature'. *Early Child Development and Care* 175 (5): 407–17. https://doi.org/10.1080/0300443042000244055.

———. 2015. 'Nutritionally "Empty" but Full of Meanings: The Socio-Cultural Significance of Birthday Cakes in Four Early Childhood Settings'. *Journal of Early Childhood Research* 13 (1): 79–92.

Alcock, Pete, and Duncan Scott. 2014. 'Voluntary and Community Sector Welfare'. In *Understanding the Mixed Economy of Welfare*, edited by Martin Powell 83–106. Bristol: The Policy Press.

Bacchi, Carol, and Susan Goodwin. 2016. *Poststructural Policy Analysis: A Guide to Practice*. New York: Palgrave Macmillan.

Boseley, Sarah. 2019. 'Leeds Becomes First UK City to Lower Its Childhood Obesity Rate'. *The Guardian*, 1 May 2019, sec. World news. http://www.theguardian.com/world/2019/may/01/leeds-becomes-first-uk-city-to-lower-its-childhood-obesity-rate.

Brewis, Alexandra. 2011. *Obesity: Cultural and Biocultural Perspectives*. New Brunswick, NJ: Rutgers University Press.

Caldeira, Teresa P. R. 2013. 'The Implosion of Modern Public Life, 2000'. In *The Anthropology of Citizenship: A Reader*, edited by Sian Lazar 229–247. Oxford: Wiley-Blackwell.

Caldwell, Melissa L. 2014. 'Epilogue: Anthropological Reflections on Critical Nutrition'. *Gastronomica: The Journal of Food and Culture* 14 (3): 67–69. https://doi.org/10.1525/gfc.2014.14.3.67.

Camps, Laura, and Tony Long. 2012. 'Origins, Purpose and Future of Sure Start Children's Centres'. *Nursing Children and Young People* 24 (1): 26–30.

Caraher, Martin, and Elizabeth Dowler. 2007. 'Food Projects in London: Lessons for Policy and Practice—A Hidden Sector and the Need for "More Unhealthy Puddings... Sometimes"'. *Health Education Journal* 66 (2): 188–205.

Centre for Longitudinal Studies. 2014. 'Child Overweight and Obesity: Initial Findings from the Millennium Chort Age 11 Survey'. London: Centre for Longitudinal Studies. www.cls.ioe.ac.uk/shared/get-file.ashx?itemtype=document&id=1952.

Childcare Act 2006. 2006. http://www.legislation.gov.uk/ukpga/2006/21/pdfs/ukpga_20060021_en.pdf.

Children's Food Trust. 2012. 'Eat Better Start Better Voluntary Food and Drink Guidelines for Early Years Settings in England – A Practical Guide'. Sheffield: Children's Food Trust. http://media.childrensfoodtrust.org.uk/2015/06/CFT_Early_Years_Guide_Interactive_Sept-12.pdf.

Clarke, Karen. 2006. 'Childhood, Parenting and Early Intervention: A Critical Examination of the Sure Start National Programme'. *Critical Social Policy* 26 (4): 699–721. https://doi.org/10.1177/0261018306068470.

Curtis, Penny, Helen Stapleton, and Allison James. 2011. 'Intergenerational Relations and the Family Food Environment in Families with a Child with Obesity'. *Annals of Human Biology* 38 (4): 429–37. https://doi.org/10.3109/03014460.2011.590530.

Department for Education. 2017. 'Statutory Framework for the Early Years Foundation Stage: Setting the Standards for Learning, Development and Care for Children from Birth to Five'. London: Department for Education. https://assets.publishing.service.gov.uk/government/uploads/system/uploads/attachment_data/file/596629/EYFS_STATUTORY_FRAMEWORK_2017.pdf.

Dermott, Esther, and Marco Pomati. 2016. '"Good" Parenting Practices: How Important Are Poverty, Education and Time Pressure?' *Sociology* 50 (1): 125–42.

Eisenberg, Merrill. 2011. 'Medical Anthropology and Public Policy'. In *A Companion to Medical Anthropology*, edited by Merrill Singer and Pamela I. Erickson 93–116. London: Blackwell Publishing Ltd.

Elias, Norbert. 1994. *The Civilizing Process*. Oxford: Blackwell Publishing Ltd.

Elliott, Victoria, and Beth Hore. 2016. '"Right Nutrition, Right Values": The Construction of Food, Youth and Morality in the UK Government 2010–2014'. *Cambridge Journal of Education* 46 (2): 177–93. https://doi.org/10.1080/0305764X.2016.1158785.

Evans, Gillian. 2017. 'Social Class and the Cultural Turn: Anthropology, Sociology and the Post-Industrial Politics of 21st Century Britain'. In *Reconfiguring the Anthropology of Britain: Ethnographic, Theoretical and Interdisciplinary Perspectives*, edited by Cathrine Degnen. The Sociological Review Monographs Series 88–106. London: SAGE Publications.

Evans, John, Laura De Pian, Emma Rich, and Brian Davies. 2011. 'Health Imperatives, Policy and the Corporeal Device: Schools, Subjectivity and Children's Health'. *Policy Futures in Education* 9 (3): 328–40. https://doi.org/10.2304/pfie.2011.9.3.328.

Evans, John, Emma Rich, and Brian Davies. 2004. 'The Emperor's New Clothes: Fat, Thin, and Overweight. The Social Fabrication of Risk and Ill Health'. *Journal of Teaching in Physical Education* 23 (4): 372–91. https://doi.org/10.1123/jtpe.23.4.372.

Faircloth, Charlotte. 2013. '"What Feels Right": Affect, Emotion, and the Limitations of Infant-Feeding Policy'. *Journal of Women, Politics & Policy* 34 (4): 345–58. https://doi.org/10.1080/1554477X.2013.835678.

Fischler, Claude. 2011. 'Commensality, Society and Culture'. *Social Science Information* 50 (3–4): 28–548.

Fitzsimons, Emla, and David Bann. 2020. 'Obesity Prevalence and Its Inequality from Childhood to Adolescence: Initial Findings from the Millennium Cohort Study Age 17 Survey'. Centre for Longitudinal Studies. https://doi.org/10.4324/9781351326520.

Fitzsimons, Emla, and Benedetta Pongiglione. 2019. 'The Impact of Maternal Employment on Children's Weight: Evidence from the UK'. *SSM - Population Health* 7 (April): 100333. https://doi.org/10.1016/j.ssmph.2018.100333.

Gibson, Sigrid, Lucy Francis, Katie Newens, and Barbara Livingstone. 2016. 'Associations between Free Sugars and Nutrient Intakes among Children and Adolescents in the UK'. *British Journal of Nutrition* 116 (07): 1265–74. https://doi.org/10.1017/S0007114516003184.

Goisis, Alice, Melissa Martinson, and Wendy Sigle. 2019. 'When Richer Doesn't Mean Thinner: Ethnicity, Socioeconomic Position, and the Risk of Child Obesity in the United Kingdom'. *Demographic Research* 41 (September): 649–78. https://doi.org/10.4054/DemRes.2019.41.23.

Goisis, Alice, Amanda Sacker, and Yvonne Kelly. 2016. 'Why Are Poorer Children at Higher Risk of Obesity and Overweight? A UK Cohort Study'. *The European Journal of Public Health* 26 (1): 7–13. https://doi.org/10.1093/eurpub/ckv219.

Greenhalgh, Susan, and Megan Carney. 2014. 'Bad Biocitizens?: Latinos and the US "Obesity Epidemic"'. *Human Organization* 73 (3): 267–76. https://doi.org/10.17730/humo.73.3.w53hh1t413038240.

Gupta, Akhil. 2012. *Red Tape Bureaucracy, Structural Violence, and Poverty in India*. Durham: Duke University Press.

Hansen, Stine Rosenlund, and Niels Heine Kristensen. 2017. 'Food for Kindergarten Children: Who Cares? Relations between Food and Care in Everyday Kindergarten Mealtime'. *Food, Culture & Society* 20 (3): 485–502. https://doi.org/10.1080/1552801 4.2017.1288783.

Hilton, Shona, Chris Patterson, and Alison Teyhan. 2012. 'Escalating Coverage of Obesity in UK Newspapers: The Evolution and Framing of the "Obesity Epidemic" From 1996 to 2010'. *Obesity* 20 (8): 1688–95. https://doi.org/10.1038/oby.2012.27.

Ingram, John S. I., Hugh L. Wright, Lucy Foster, Timothy Aldred, David Barling, Tim G. Benton, Paul M. Berryman, et al. 2013. 'Priority Research Questions for the UK Food System'. *Food Security* 5 (5): 617–36. https://doi.org/10.1007/s12571-013-0294-4.

Kelly, Aaron S., and Stephen R. Daniels. 2017. 'Rethinking the Use of Body Mass Index z-Score in Children and Adolescents with Severe Obesity: Time to Kick It to the Curb?' *The Journal of Pediatrics* 188 (September): 7–8. https://doi.org/10.1016/j.jpeds.2017.05.003.

Lambert, Michael. 2019. 'Between "Families in Trouble" and "Children at Risk": Historicising "Troubled Family" Policy in England since 1945'. *Children & Society* 33 (1): 82–91. https://doi.org/10.1111/chso.12309.

Lee, Nick, and Johanna Motzkau. 2011. 'Navigating the Bio-Politics of Childhood'. *Childhood* 18 (1): 7–19. https://doi.org/10.1177/0907568210371526.

Lemke, Thomas. 2001. '"The Birth of Bio-Politics": Michel Foucault's Lecture at the Collège de France on Neo-Liberal Governmentality'. *Economy and Society* 30 (2): 190–207. https://doi.org/10.1080/03085140120042271.

Lister, Ruth. 2008. 'Unpacking Children's Citizenship'. In *Children and Citizenship*, edited by Antonella Invernizzi and Jane Williams 9–19. London: SAGE Publications.

Macvarish, Jan. 2014. 'The Politics of Parenting'. In *Parenting Culture Studies*, edited by Ellie Lee, Jennie Bristow, Charlotte Faircloth, and Jan Macvarish. Basingstoke: Palgrave Macmillan.

Maher, JaneMaree, Fraser, Suzanne, and Lindsay, Jo. 2010. 'Between Provisioning and Consuming?: Children, Mothers and "Childhood Obesity"'. *Health Sociology Review* 19 (3): 304–16.

Moffat, Tina. 2010. 'The "Childhood Obesity Epidemic": Health Crisis or Social Construction?' *Medical Anthropology Quarterly* 24 (1): 1–21. https://doi.org/10.1111/j.1548-1387.2010.01082.x.

Mol, Annemarie. 2008. *The Logic of Care: Health and the Problem of Patient Choice*. London: Routledge.

Moss, Peter, and Pat Petrie. 2000. *From Children's Services to Children's Spaces*. London: Routledge/Falmer.

Mucavele, Patricia, Laura Sharp, Claire Wall, and Jo Nicholas. 2014. 'Children's Food Trust "Eat Better, Start Better" Programme: Outcomes and Recommendations'. *Perspectives in Public Health* 134 (2): 67–69. https://doi.org/10.1177/1757913914523910.

Murphy, Elizabeth. 2000. 'Risk, Responsibility and Rhetoric in Infant Feeding'. *Journal of Contemporary Ethnography* 29 (3): 291–325.

National Statistics. 2022. 'National Child Measurement Programme, England, 2021/22 School Year'. NDRS. 3 November 2022. https://digital.nhs.uk/data-and-information/publications/statistical/national-child-measurement-programme/2021-22-school-year.

Nursery World. 2017. 'Children's Food Trust to Close'. *Nursery World* (blog). 21 July 2017. https://www.nurseryworld.co.uk/nursery-world/news/1161785/childrens-food-trust-to-close.

O'Connell, Rebecca, and Julia Brannen. 2016. *Food, Families and Work*. London: Bloomsbury.

O'Connell, Rebecca, Charlie Owen, Matt Padley, Antonia Simon, and Julia Brannen. 2018. 'Which Types of Family Are at Risk of Food Poverty in the UK? A Relative Deprivation

Approach'. *Social Policy and Society*, February, 1–18. https://doi.org/10.1017/S1474746418000015.

Pearce, Anna, Steven Hope, Lucy Griffiths, Mario Cortina-Borja, Catherine Chittleborough, and Catherine Law. 2019. 'What If All Children Achieved WHO Recommendations on Physical Activity? Estimating the Impact on Socioeconomic Inequalities in Childhood Overweight in the UK Millennium Cohort Study'. *International Journal of Epidemiology* 48 (1): 134–47. https://doi.org/10.1093/ije/dyy267.

Penn, Helen. 2007. 'Childcare Market Management: How the United Kingdom Government Has Reshaped Its Role in Developing Early Childhood Education and Care'. *Contemporary Issues in Early Childhood* 8 (3): 192–207. https://doi.org/10.2304/ciec.2007.8.3.192.

Perkins, Clare, and Eustace DeSousa. 2018. 'Trends in Childhood Height and Weight, and Socioeconomic Inequalities'. *The Lancet Public Health* 3 (4): e160–61. https://doi.org/10.1016/S2468-2667(18)30050-1.

Petersen, Alan, and Deborah Lupton. 1996. *The New Public Health: Health and Self in the Age of Risk*. London: SAGE Publications.

Power, Michael. 1999. *The Audit Society: Rituals of Verification*. Oxford: Oxford University Press.

Public Health England, Victoria Targett, and Rachel Allen. 2015. 'Sugar Reduction: The Evidence for Action.' London: Public Health England. https://www.gov.uk/government/uploads/system/uploads/attachment_data/file/470179/Sugar_reduction_The_evidence_for_action.pdf.

Qvortrup, Jens. 2005. 'Varieties of Childhood'. In *Studies in Modern Childhood: Society, Agency, Culture*, edited by Jens Qvortrup, 1–20. Basingstoke: Palgrave Macmillan.

Rees, Rebecca, Kathryn Oliver, Jenny Woodman, and James Thomas. 2011. 'The Views of Young Children in the UK about Obesity, Body Size, Shape and Weight: A Systematic Review'. *BMC Public Health* 11 (1). https://doi.org/10.1186/1471-2458-11-188.

Roberts, Kim. 2015. 'Growing Up Not out: The HENRY Approach to Preventing Childhood Obesity'. *British Journal of Obesity* 1 (3): 87–92.

Rose, Nikolas. 1996. 'Governing "Advanced" Liberal Democracies'. In *Foucault and Political Reason. Liberalism, Neo-Liberalism and Rationalities of Government*, edited by Andrew Barry, Thomas Osborne, and Nikolas Rose 37–64. London: Routledge.

Rose, Nikolas, and Filippa Lentzos. 2017. 'Making Us Resilient: Responsible Citizens for Uncertain Times'. In *Competing Responsibilities: The Ethics and Politics of Contemporary Life*, edited by Susanna Trnka and Catherine Trundle 27–48. Durham: Duke University Press.

Rougeaux, Emeline, Steven Hope, Catherine Law, and Anna Pearce. 2017. 'Have Health Inequalities Changed during Childhood in the New Labour Generation? Findings from the UK Millennium Cohort Study'. *BMJ Open* 7 (1): e012868. https://doi.org/10.1136/bmjopen-2016-012868.

Sayer, Andrew. 2017. 'Responding to the Troubled Families Programme: Framing the Injuries of Inequality'. *Social Policy and Society* 16 (01): 155–64. https://doi.org/10.1017/S1474746416000373.

Schrecker, Ted. 2017. 'Was Mackenbach Right? Towards a Practical Political Science of Redistribution and Health Inequalities'. *Health & Place* 46 (July): 293–99. https://doi.org/10.1016/j.healthplace.2017.06.007.

Scientific Advisory Committee on Nutrition. 2015. *Carbohydrates and Health*. London: Public Health England.

Shore, Cris. 2017. 'Audit Culture and the Politics of Responsibility: Beyond Neoliberal Responsibilization?' In *Competing Responsibilities: The Ethics and Politics of Contemporary Life*, edited by Susanna Trnka and Catherine Trundle 96–117. Durham: Duke University Press.

Shore, Cris, and Susan Wright. 1997. 'Policy: A New Field of Anthropology'. In *Anthropology of Policy: Critical Perspectives on Governance and Power*, edited by Cris Shore and Susan Wright. London: Routlegde.

Stats Team, NHS Digital. 2018. 'National Child Measurement Programme: England, 2017/ 18 School Year'. London: The Health and Social Innovation Centre. https://digital.nhs.uk/ data-and-information/publications/statistical/national-child-measurement-programme/ 2017-18-school-year#summary.

Throsby, Karen. 2018. 'Giving Up Sugar and the Inequalities of Abstinence'. *Sociology of Health & Illness* 40 (6): 954–68. https://doi.org/10.1111/1467-9566.12734.

Times, Toby McDonald | The Sunday. 2019. 'Nice Work, Mum: You've Turned Me into a Lazy Lardy'. *The Times*, 9 March 2019, sec. News. https://www.thetimes.co.uk/article/ nice-work-mum-youve-turned-me-into-a-lazy-lardy-5x98xzrn6.

Tisdall, E. Kay M., and Samantha Punch. 2012. 'Not so "New"? Looking Critically at Childhood Studies'. *Children's Geographies* 10 (3): 249–64. https://doi.org/10.1080/14 733285.2012.693376.

Trnka, Susanna, and Catherine Trundle. 2014. 'Competing Responsibilities: Moving Beyond Neoliberal Responsibilisation'. *Anthropological Forum* 24 (2): 136–53. https://doi.org/1 0.1080/00664677.2013.879051.

Ulijaszek, Stanley J., and Amy K. McLennan. 2016. 'Framing Obesity in UK Policy from the Blair Years, 1997-2015: The Persistence of Individualistic Approaches despite Overwhelming Evidence of Societal and Economic Factors, and the Need for Collective Responsibility'. *Obesity Reviews* 17 (5): 397–411. https://doi.org/10.1111/obr.12386.

Vander Schee, Carolyn. 2009. 'Fruit, Vegetables, Fatness, and Foucault: Governing Students and Their Families through School Health Policy'. *Journal of Education Policy* 24 (5): 557–74. https://doi.org/10.1080/02680930902823047.

Warin, Megan, Karen Turner, Vivienne Moore, and Michael Davies. 2008. 'Bodies, Mothers and Identities: Rethinking Obesity and the BMI'. *Sociology of Health & Illness* 30 (1): 97–111. https://doi.org/10.1111/j.1467-9566.2007.01029.x.

Yates-Doerr, Emily. 2015. *The Weight of Obesity : Hunger and Global Health in Postwar Guatemala*. Oakland, California: University of California Press.

2 The food industry and its contradictions

Based on existing literature (Atkins 2005; MacMillan, Dowler, and Archard 2006; Lang and Rayner 2010; Wiley 2011; Lang and Barling 2013; O'Connell and Brannen 2016) and my own empirical data, this chapter will unpack some of the interactions between the state and food industry, showing the contradictions that can arise when marketed food products are included in policy and public health encounters, adding complexity to questions around whose responsibility it is to provide 'good' food to children, explored in Chapter 1. Still focusing on the 'problems' of obesity and high sugar intake (discussed in the previous chapter), the topic of marketing food to children will be explored, drawing from conversations I had with parents at Ladybird. These exchanges pointed to the value and meanings attributed to 'children's food' – as a category that is separate to that of 'adult food.' Drawing from scholars such as James (1998); Curtis, James, and Ellis (2010); and Patico and Lozada (2015), the chapter will show how the food industry capitalises on these distinctive qualities assigned to children's food, but also on the fact that one of the few domains where children can exert a higher degree of autonomy (especially the very young) is food choice.

Yet, it is not only the unique elements of 'children's food' that play a part in shaping food industry strategies, but so is adopting the language of public health – in this way, food products marketed to children can simultaneously appeal to young consumers as well as the adults who feed them. The role that the food industry plays in determining people's diets, and its interaction with state policy, will thus be assessed. Following from Chapter 1, which explored how the notions of 'responsibility' and 'choice' are operationalised in policy, and drawing from my own ethnographic material, I will examine how parents are still widely held as solely responsible for determining their children's diets. This becomes particularly contentious when industrialised food products become part of public health and family policy interventions that focus on teaching people how to read food labels and make choices based on this (sometimes arbitrary) knowledge, as I will show through parents' accounts and my own observations of food education initiatives. Families and children are often told that they should be suspicious of industrialised food products, yet the guidelines and messaging that these contain (e.g. on packaging) are promoted as methods that can help people make 'healthy choices.' This is especially difficult, however, when the food industry co-opts the language

DOI: 10.4324/9781003297642-3

of public health to sell products. An emphasis on "numbers and accounting metaphors" (Caldwell 2014, 68) in dietary guidelines, which present 'choices' as easier to make, further reinforces the narrative of individual responsibility inherent in policy and mainstream discourses. Missing from these paradigms are people's lived experience and children's voices, obscuring the key role that food plays in shaping relations of care.

Critiques of the food industry

The food industry's role in determining food supply and people's diets has been less well documented in the U.K. compared to some of the work conducted in the United States (e.g. Wiley 2011; Nestle 2013). Nonetheless, particularly for the case of 'children's food,' studies have been carried out to explore the motivations that the state and the food industry have had in promoting certain food products and policies. Atkins, for instance, has questioned whether the provision of milk to school children during the 1950s and 1960s in Britain was a policy propelled by the aim of improving children's health, or whether it was a measure to boost the British agricultural sector and to 'train' children "to become loyal adult consumers" (2005, 58). This is echoed by Wiley for the U.S. context, who proposes that there is a blurred understanding of 'growth' in relation to milk production and consumption – it brings together the State's commitment to grow the agricultural sector with a concern for sustaining children's health and growth (2014, 120).

As well as raising questions about whose interests are being prioritised and promoted when certain food products are marketed as 'good' for children, the impact this has in creating moralised notions of 'healthy food' also needs to be explored. Milk, in particular, continues to be considered central to children's growth and development in the U.K., as in many other countries (Wiley 2014). Yet, as explored in Chapter 1, what is 'good' or 'healthy' in policy and mainstream discourse (and what is included and excluded in these definitions) is decided by the authoritative voices within the children's food policy and public health arenas. MacMillan, Dowler, and Archard (2006) have discussed who are the different actors that are held responsible for children's diets in the U.K. They point out that what children consume outside of the home environment has historically received less attention:

> Public opinion that parents *ought to be* responsible for the diets of their children…is commonly reported as the opinion that parents *are* responsible for children's diets…Indeed, as parental control over children's diets has diminished, the ethical and legal language for describing the relationship of parents to children has shifted from that of parental rights over children to parental duties of care. If parents discharge this duty by ensuring adequate home diets, can they also reasonably be held responsible for what their children eat outside the home? What are the responsibilities of food companies acting *in loco parentis*?
>
> (2006, 240, original emphasis)

Further, these authors assess whether food corporations, and those who regulate the distribution of 'bad' foods in the market, are to be held equally, or more or less, accountable if children develop unhealthy eating habits (ibid.). They also discuss the topic of 'food environments,' and the extent to which children have autonomy in making decisions about their diets within these environments (ibid., 241). They conclude that children's food policies can be reimagined so that they can support and encourage their autonomy, but that this cannot be done unless their voices are also included in the policymaking process (ibid.). This is a particularly urgent point to think about when children's autonomy and agency flourishes and is exercised where there are structures in place that potentially negatively impact their well-being (such as the U.K.'s over-industrialised food system).

The question of children's engagement with the food industry is thus an important one to consider, even in the context of the early years. This is one of the only domains where infants and young children have more control over their daily lives and can contest adults' attempts to regulate their behaviour (O'Connell 2010, 573). However, as alluded to above, the notion of children's autonomy should be assessed carefully when considering how these preferences are shaped by the food environment, and when products are marketed specifically to children. As O'Connell and Brannen suggest, not all parents are equally able to counteract the influence of the food industry on their children's dietary choices (2016, 98). Curtis, James, and Ellis (2010) point to the 'disruptive' role that foods advertised and sold to children plays. 'Children's food' disrupt social norms, as these products are often to be consumed outside of the home and in 'non-traditional' mealtime settings, but are also disruptive in nutritional terms, since 'children's food' is often considered unhealthy by adults. This is in line with an early argument posed by James (1998), who contends that, in addition to fostering children's autonomy and independence, 'junk' foods, sweets, and foods marketed specifically as 'children's food' play a central part in creating children's cultures, often helping to make a clear separation between the world of adults and their own. James argues that the food industry capitalises on these distinctive features of 'children's food,' making them conspicuous in products' "names, their colours, the sensations they induce, their presentation and the descriptions of their contents" (ibid., 397), in addition to making these foods suitable for the way in which, and circumstances when, children consume them (e.g. when out and about together). Patico and Lozada have similarly shown that food marketing strategies aimed at children focus on the emotional dimension of sharing food with peers, and depict food consumption in the 'non-traditional' settings (2015, 208) which James (1998) discusses as one of the elements that sets 'children's foods' apart from the adult world.

These things considered, the question of food marketing aimed at children was thus a major concern that parents brought up in conversations with me, and which also emerged in the interactions that took place at some of the local interventions that I took part in during my fieldwork. Several parents spoke of their young children's abilities to recognise brands, and expressed being concerned about both the appeal and 'addictiveness' of the foods that their children knew and liked. This came up during a focused group discussion with three mothers whose children attended Ladybird nursery:

OLGA: [...] someone has introduced [my daughter] to Ribena,[1] so she drags me
to the shop for Ribena.

JANE: Oh no, that's awful, Ribena! No, don't give her Ribena...

OLGA: I hate that drink. But she cries, if we pass the shop on the way home and
we don't go in.

JANE: She cries?

OLGA: She knows, I'm like, "OK, I'll get you one." On the way home the other
day we passed the shop, and she couldn't find the blackcurrant one, on
the shelf there was only the strawberry one, and she comes from the shelf
"Ahhh" [crying sounds] crying, I'm like, "Why are you crying?" and
she's like, "Because there is no Ribena left!"
[laughter]

JANE: It's all the sugar, isn't it, it's addiction to sugar.

BETTY: Yeah...

This account exemplifies the limitations of viewing parents as solely capable to
shape children's eating, challenging the view that adults can impact children's
practices in a unidirectional and imposing manner (Curtis, Stapleton, and James
2011, 435). Children, even at a young age, can exert authority in powerful ways,
like Olga's daughter. Furthermore, as Albon argues, there is a wide net of relationships, situations, and places that affect children's diets (2007, 257), and there is
ample evidence to suggest that even young children can recognise brands and shape
their preferences in relation to them (e.g. Marshall 2005; Gram 2015). Nonetheless,
also among parents, the current crisis rhetoric around children's high sugar intake
(explored in Chapter 1) muddies perceptions about who is responsible for children's diets. In the conversation with mothers above, 'sugar addiction' is identified
as one of the issues that leads Olga's daughter to regularly request Ribena, shifting
focus from the food environment.

Yet, for the most part, the pervasiveness of food advertising and fast-food
outlets was experienced as difficult and anxiety-inducing by many of the parents I
spoke to. Worries around the availability of sugary drinks and fast-food chains like
McDonald's were raised during a home interview with Jane and her four-year-old
daughter Luisa:

*Jane talks to me about the times she and Luisa have travelled to Mexico to
visit family, telling me about the differences between what she and Luisa eat
when they are there compared to when they are in London. She particularly
laments that giving fizzy, sugary drinks to children is such common practice
in Mexico, and how difficult she finds refusing them to Luisa when they come
back to London, even though she knows limiting her sugar intake is what is
best for her. Luisa interjects during this exchange:*

LUISA: My dad eats cow's eyeballs!

JANE: Yes, in tacos, quite Mexican...but you see, Luisa is quite interested in
McDonald's...

LUISA: But I don't eat it. I always see it…
JANE: There's just adverts everywhere…and it's not just adverts, it's in rubbish bins, it's people eating it, it's just everywhere!
LUISA: I've got a good eye!
JANE: [laughs] Yes you've got a good eye to see all these things!
LUISA: I always see it! I say, look there's a McDonald's poster over there! Like when I'm on the bus or on the way to school. I found an old McDonald's on the road…
JANE: An old wrapper didn't you…?
LUISA: Yes!

This exchange again points to the ubiquity of marketed food products in families' and children's daily lives, the awareness that children have of brands (even at a young age), and how their curiosity and preferences are formed in relation to these. Yet, in addition to children's varied ways of engaging with and responding to the food industry, Jane's comments on people giving sugary drinks to children as common practice in Mexico also points to a further contradiction related to how 'children's food' is thought of. As alluded to in this chapter so far, both by public health and parents' standards, 'children's food' is often considered unhealthy. However, giving these foods to children is also a way in which adults enact care towards them. Like Jane's accounts of visiting family in Mexico, during the focus group discussion quoted above, Olga shared:

> *[…] if my mum comes [to visit us], she spoils [my daughter] with sweets, and crisps, and all those sugary drinks.*

In a home interview I carried out with Adriana, another woman whose child attended Ladybird, she lamented her husband's tendency to give their daughter sugary foods as a reward for 'good behaviour':

> *When [our daughter] behaves well he will reward her that way, he will give her a sweet […] I try to reward her in other ways, I always tell her, 'If you behave we can watch a film, or we can go to the park,' but I never give her sweets or ice-cream as a reward…only her father [does].* [2]

Whilst it is evidently frustrating for parents when other adults influence their children's eating practices in a way that is negatively perceived, these accounts do suggest that when adults give children 'junk' foods they are 'spoiling' or 'treating' them – it is a way to show love and care. This contested quality of 'children's food,' as simultaneously unhealthy and as a vehicle through which care is enacted, is also documented by Albon (2005, 2015), who highlights that the symbolic meaning of sugary foods (as expressions of care) very often outweighs their 'nutritional emptiness.'

Taking this into account, and children's engagement with the food industry (e.g. when visiting shops and via marketing campaigns), policy efforts to address childhood obesity and high sugar intake through market-based solutions have been met with some scepticism by professionals and scholars alike. Marion Nestle has pointed out, for example, that efforts to restrict or regulate what is produced, marketed, and sold by large corporations have largely been futile: "Advice to restrict any food invariably distresses its producers and sellers; these lobby relentlessly – and often successfully – for retraction" (2006, 564). Similarly, media analysis by Elliott-Green et al. (2016) has shown some of the challenges that policymakers will face when proposing market-based solutions to reduce high sugar intakes. When comparing public health versus industry messaging of sugar-sweetened beverages (SSBs) in mainstream media, Elliott-Green et al. found that, "Although a largely unified approach presented from Action on Sugar, WHO and public health officials was presented to the media, this largely failed to penetrate large sections of the British press, with most articles neglecting to control SSBs" (2016, 7). Importantly, they also assess industry responses to the newly proposed regulations on SSBs and media coverage, arguing that similar to some of the strategies adopted by the tobacco industry, food corporations promote fitness and exercise, or market fat-free or sugar-free versions of their products as a way to highlight individual responsibility and choice, simultaneously promoting an image of social corporate responsibility (ibid.). In this way, the food industry both capitalises on children's autonomy and agency as described above, but also on the public health guidelines and messaging that matter to adults.

Corporate interests can often also feed on scientific uncertainties. In the Danish context, Vallgårda et al. (2015) showed that one of the causes that led to the failure of the tax on saturated fats was health experts' scepticism that the tax would have significant, if any, effects on people's health (2015, 224–25), and further questioned whether the tax would actually lead to healthier foods entering the market or if less healthy products would be sold instead (ibid., 224). The authors show that key stakeholders in the agricultural and dairy industries backed research and the dissemination of findings that raised these concerns about the health outcomes of the tax and, in doing so, very effectively lobbied against it (ibid., 225). By a similar token, Moffat has argued that the 'problems' of childhood obesity and high sugar intake have even been seen by many corporations in the United States as an opportunity for financial gain: "profiting from ill health is not unique to the obesity epidemic and is part and parcel of a wider capitalistic health care system" (2010, 8). Indeed, Britain is not far behind in this regard.

The food industry and its contradictions

The 'Food Matters Live' conference ended today. These last two days have given me a close insight into the multiple contradictions that arise when discussing any issues related to children's food policy. The event brought together a wide range of public health and policy experts on 'crisis' topics (such as childhood obesity) to discuss possible approaches to solving these issues – at the same time that we were also surrounded by food industry representatives showcasing their products. It seems – counterintuitively – that these 'crises' are currently being used by many companies as marketing opportunities – fieldnotes, November 2016.

Holding the food industry accountable for people's diets in the context of advanced liberalism is difficult. As Ulijaszek and McLennan have noted for the matter of obesity:

> Obesity policymaking is not neutral; it is a process that takes place within societies. Societies, in turn, have specific social values, norms and power hierarchies, which vary between and within nations, and across time. The people involved in policymaking processes have particular backgrounds, ideologies and interrelations, all of which influence how they act. And the pressures that shape policymaking and government reporting frequently go unreported or even unnoticed. Policies which emerge reflect the landscape of policymakers, advisors, political pressures and values, as much – if not more – than the landscape of evidence. *The power position of industry and those supported by it…remains largely unchallenged; in this case, individualistic framing offers the path of least resistance.*
>
> (2016, 409, own emphasis)

These were very much my impressions after I attended the 'Food Matters Live' conference held in London in November 2016. The event brought together some of the foremost experts in public health and food policy to put forward solutions to some of the challenges being faced by the U.K. food system and its consumers. Whilst on the one hand raising concern for the changes in the kind of products available to us in a highly industrialised food system, the emphasis on solutions remained largely individualistic. This seemed fitting. Outside the conference rooms where these discussions were unfolding, hundreds of product stalls were lined up with different kinds of 'healthy' foods available to be sampled. Many of these were labelled as low-sugar, low-fat, zero-calorie foods. The selling points were clear, and very much a response to the 'problems' of obesity and high sugar intake described in official discourse. Making these products available also plays into the narrative of 'choice' and individual responsibility explored thus far; it is up to consumers to make the 'right' choices in relation to food, and often these 'choices' are presented as easy to make if food products are labelled as healthy.

'Food Matters Live' seemed overwhelming to me, because of the wide range of sectors represented by the event participants, and the magnitude of the issues covered. Nonetheless, the contradictions I noted during those days were the very ones I was also observing in the field. For example, parents who were targeted for interventions around food and eating were being encouraged to learn how to read food labels to avoid 'bad' foods for their children.[3]

This approach was central in one of the Health, Exercise and Nutrition for the Really Young (HENRY)[4] (Roberts 2015) sessions offered to parents at a children's centre in the borough where I carried out fieldwork. The session involved a number of interactive tasks on the topic of nutrition, including an activity focused on reading food labels. In my fieldnotes from that day, I noted some of the contradictions that arose during this activity:

> One of the parents brought some packets of the different food items that she gives to her baby, to check their labels with the rest of the group (this included a multipack of Heinz-brand fruit and vegetable pots, some biscuits suitable for babies, and Aptamil-brand muesli). She keeps repeating, "There's a lot on the list," both for the foods she brought and the empty food packet the session leader gave her for the activity. The woman then reveals the sugar content in the muesli she brought with disapproval; the rest of the group also seems quite shocked, since this is a product marketed specifically for young infants, who should not be having high doses of refined sugars. The HENRY instructor inspects the label and determines the sugar is derived from the dried fruits mixed in the muesli, so reassures the woman who brought the packet that she shouldn't worry. After this, a discussion about the merits and drawbacks of this particular brand of products ensues – fieldnotes, March 2017.

Again, the potential for 'good' foods to become 'bad' was evident during this interaction at the HENRY session. In the case of processed foods, or products marketed as 'good' for children, this can become even more of a complicated domain to navigate for parents (Isaacs, Neve, and Hawkes 2022), and one in which the moral dimensions of food and parenting practices are particularly perceptible. This tension was evident during another focused group discussion I conducted with three mothers:

VIVIAN: I remember going to 'soft play' at [another] children's centre, and you can bring your own snacks, so I would take some snacks. And I remember seeing some mums would come with whole…tupperwares full of vegetables that all their kids would happily be eating, raw vegetables, and I'd be like, wow, how did you get them to do that? […] I discovered that things like dried apricots, and dried figs, and dried prunes…I used to carry them as snacks, yeah, and I discovered that they're a total no-no when I went to take [my son] to the dentist the first time, and she said no, you might as well give him a packet of Haribos [candy]. And then I used to take him to some of the drop-ins at other children's centres… and uhm…one of the drop-ins mentioned that to the parents, but others didn't […] And not really knowing, you get all those snacks, all those snacks you get in the shops, those bear fruit loop things…
STACEY: Oh yeah, the 'Yo-Yo' [brand].
VIVIAN: Yeah, there's so many things when you go into the shops that are just for the kids and toddlers, and the way they are packaged, they don't look like candy, they look like healthy and good, and it's got the five-a-day [label], and you think "Oh yeah, ok," and then…actually, they're full of sugar. And you don't know about that, so then you see some parents giving them, just like a whole fruit loop to their four-year-old, and…I don't know, I don't really know, is that OK, is that not OK?

The anxieties that parents expressed during the HENRY session and during the focus group discussion evidence how the food industry contributes to the contested nature of, and confusion around, what constitutes 'good' food for children. Yet, these interactions also point to the added difficulties that arise alongside the increasing appearance of 'food pedagogies' (Flowers and Swan 2016) across the world.[5] Flowers and Swan coined this term to describe the rise of education initiatives about food and diet, which have emerged together with new groups of experts that communicate knowledge and information about food to the public, with children and families being particularly targeted by these initiatives (ibid., 22).

Across the borough where I conducted fieldwork, childcare practitioners and other staff members responsible for feeding children also took part in food education sessions and courses, some of which took a similar approach to that of the HENRY session described above in using food packaging. One of these courses, attended by some of the staff at Ladybird, was intended to equip practitioners with the knowledge and skills outlined in the Children's Food Trust's 'Eat Better Start Better' (EBSB) framework (Children's Food Trust 2012).[6] In the fieldnotes from that day I noted:

The final activity in today's session is about understanding food labels. We are given some cards explaining what is the purpose of all the different food labels on food packaging (like an ingredients list or the red, yellow, green labels indicating recommended daily intakes). We are then made to analyse different food packages following these guidelines. Everyone in the room takes turns sharing whether the package we got is 'healthy' or not, according to the food labels guidelines we discussed before. The last person to speak is holding a snack bar from a popular vegan brand, generally marketed as a healthy option. Yet, to the participant, the product seemed 'unhealthy' because all the contents (sugar, fat, etc.) were marked by red bubbles (indicating levels higher than the daily recommended daily intake) – fieldnotes, March 2017.

The potential for 'good' foods to become 'bad' was thus also present in professional settings. In all the interactions and exchanges described above, some of the limitations of policy and public health responses to the pressures people face when navigating the U.K.'s food system are evident. It is apparent that widening knowledge and skills can be problematic when public health messaging is used as a marketing strategy by the food industry. By co-opting the notion of 'goodness' into its domain, the food industry also further validates the centrality of individual responsibility that predominates under advanced liberalism, and which is reproduced on the ground through interventions such as the HENRY or EBSB approaches. Mol's critique of this paradigm is not only that it creates "cold and distanced relations" (2008, 18) – between people, and also between the public and decision-makers – but that it frames the act of 'choosing' as momentary and finite (and lonely), as separate from the wide range of other conditions and social circumstances that people confront and navigate daily, collectively rather than as individuals. As O'Connell and

Brannen have argued, policy should move beyond individualistic, nutrition-driven approaches to promote responses that focus on dietary education, but equally on creating stricter regulations for the food industry (2016, 150). Similarly, others have pointed to the importance of adequately considering people's lived experience when drafting food policy (Centre for Food Policy 2018; Neve et al. 2021).

And indeed, it does appear that a shift is happening within policy discourse, where the structural factors that impact people's diets (including the role of the food industry) are increasingly being considered. Public Health England's 'Sugar Reduction Strategy' (Public Health England 2015) and the HENRY approach, which were examined in Chapter 1, do take the 'obesogenic environment' into consideration within their frameworks. Headlines about children's nutrition and diets have also increasingly drawn attention to the contradictions that parents face when buying food for their children: "Parents being misled over kids' snacks, says child health expert," the BBC reported (*BBC News* 2019). Nonetheless, within the policies examined in Chapter 1, and in these media narratives, it is still consumers that are being held responsible for avoiding these unhealthy foods, as explained by the BBC:

> Researcher Dr Ada Garcia told the BBC: 'At the moment some companies are using health messaging to make products more attractive to people, but they do not always live up to those claims. It is important parents don't look at the claims in isolation but look at all the ingredients on the pack and judge the whole quality of the food.'

> (ibid.)

Thus, new framings of 'problems' related to children's food and eating will continue to be limited if based on the premise that individual choice is a central determinant of health outcomes. This is particularly disadvantageous to socioeconomically vulnerable groups, as the price of fresh, more nutritious, food rises, and that of processed foods (higher in sugar, saturated fat, and salt content) remains much more widely affordable (e.g. Jones et al. 2014; Overseas Development Institute (ODI) 2015). The reality of the increasing cost of food, paired to children's engagement with the food industry (and the food industry's skilfulness to make products attractive to children), are not always adequately considered in nutrition-driven policy responses. The role that the food industry plays in shaping children's diets adds an additional layer of complexity to the questions about responsibility explored in Chapter 1. 'Choice,' as has been shown throughout this chapter, is not linear or just contingent on the amount of information people have available to them, or their ability to make sense of this knowledge. As Isaacs and colleagues have also argued, in relation to low-income families' food shopping practices, there are a multitude of other factors that impact people's food choices, from accessibility and convenience of shops' locations, to affordability, to the social relations that are formed and maintained through shopping activities (Isaacs et al. 2022). And, as I have also shown, children (even the very young) are often involved in all of these practices; Isaacs et al. found, too, that parents in their study were regularly unable (and sometimes unwilling) to limit their children's access and consumption of 'aggressively marketed' foods (ibid., 6).

These final reflections help us return to the argument outlined above around the contested nature of 'children's food' as both unhealthy and as an expression of care. Caring through food, even when this involves dietary transgressions, is often as (or more) important than adhering to dietary guidelines, or following market-based incentives to reduce consumption of these goods. The tension between the universalism of policy and the particularism of care is again evident; in the context of institutionalised childcare, caring through food within the policy and food industry context that I have described provides further insight of how this tension manifests in the everyday lives of children and adults. This will be unpacked at length in the following chapter.

Notes

1 Popular brand of fruit juice in the U.K., made from fruit concentrate.
2 Own translation from Spanish.
3 This approach followed by official actors will be explored at length in Chapter 5.
4 'The HENRY Approach to Preventing Childhood Obesity' was introduced and discussed in detail in Chapter 1.
5 Food pedagogies and the use of food as a 'pedagogical tool' will be discussed at length in the following chapter.
6 The 'Eat Better Start Better' framework was introduced and discussed at length in Chapter 1.

References

Albon, Deborah. 2005. 'Approaches to the Study of Children, Food and Sweet Eating: A Review of the Literature'. *Early Child Development and Care* 175 (5): 407–17. https://doi.org/10.1080/0300443042000244055.

———. 2015. 'Nutritionally "Empty" but Full of Meanings: The Socio-Cultural Significance of Birthday Cakes in Four Early Childhood Settings'. *Journal of Early Childhood Research* 13 (1): 79–92.

Atkins, Peter J. 2005. 'Fattening Children or Fattening Farmers? School Milk in Britain, 1921–1941'. *The Economic History Review* 58 (1): 57–78.

BBC News. 2019. 'Parents "Being Misled over Kids" Snacks"', 5 April 2019, sec. Health. https://www.bbc.com/news/health-47791788.

Caldwell, Melissa L. 2014. 'Epilogue: Anthropological Reflections on Critical Nutrition'. *Gastronomica: The Journal of Food and Culture* 14 (3): 67–69. https://doi.org/10.1525/gfc.2014.14.3.67.

Centre for Food Policy. 2018. *How Can Evidence of Lived Experience Make Food Policy More Effective and Equitable in Addressing Major Food System Challenges? Report of the City Food Symposium 2018*. London: Centre for Food Policy.

Children's Food Trust. 2012. 'Eat Better Start Better Voluntary Food and Drink Guidelines for Early Years Settings in England – A Practical Guide'. Sheffield: Children's Food Trust. http://media.childrensfoodtrust.org.uk/2015/06/CFT_Early_Years_Guide_Interactive_Sept-12.pdf.

Curtis, Penny, Allison James, and Katie Ellis. 2010. 'Children's Snacking, Children's Food: Food Moralities and Family Life'. *Children's Geographies* 8 (3): 291–302. https://doi.org /10.1080/14733285.2010.494870.

Curtis, Penny, Helen Stapleton, and Allison James. 2011. 'Intergenerational Relations and the Family Food Environment in Families with a Child with Obesity'. *Annals of Human Biology* 38 (4): 429–37. https://doi.org/10.3109/03014460.2011.590530.

Elliott-Green, Alex, Lirije Hyseni, Ffion Lloyd-Williams, Helen Bromley, and Simon Capewell. 2016. 'Sugar-Sweetened Beverages Coverage in the British Media: An Analysis of Public Health Advocacy Versus Pro-Industry Messaging'. *BMJ Open* 6 (7): e011295. https://doi.org/10.1136/bmjopen-2016-011295.

Flowers, Rick, and Elaine Swan, eds. 2016. *Food Pedagogies*. London: Routledge.

Gram, Malene. 2015. 'Buying Food for the Family: Negotiations in Parent/Child Supermarket Shopping: An Observational Study from Denmark and the United States'. *Journal of Contemporary Ethnography* 44 (2): 169–95. https://doi.org/10.1177/0891241614533125.

Isaacs, Anna, Joel Halligan, Kimberley Neve, and Corinna Hawkes. 2022. 'From Healthy Food Environments to Healthy Wellbeing Environments: Policy Insights from a Focused Ethnography with Low-Income Parents' in England'. *Health & Place* 77 (September): 102862. https://doi.org/10.1016/j.healthplace.2022.102862.

Isaacs, Anna, Kimberley Neve, and Corinna Hawkes. 2022. 'Why Do Parents Use Packaged Infant Foods When Starting Complementary Feeding? Findings from Phase One of a Longitudinal Qualitative Study'. *BMC Public Health* 22 (1): 2328. https://doi. org/10.1186/s12889-022-14637-0.

James, Allison. 1998. 'Confections, Concoctions and Conceptions'. In *The Children's Culture Reader*, edited by Henry Jenkins, 394–305. New York: New York University Press.

Jones, Nicholas R. V., Annalijn I. Conklin, Marc Suhrcke, and Pablo Monsivais. 2014. 'The Growing Price Gap between More and Less Healthy Foods: Analysis of a Novel Longitudinal UK Dataset'. Edited by Harry Zhang. *PLoS ONE* 9 (10): 1–7. https://doi. org/10.1371/journal.pone.0109343.

Lang, Tim, and David Barling. 2013. 'UK Food Policy: Can We Get It on the Right Track?' *Food Ethics* 8 (3): 4–7.

Lang, Tim, and Geof Rayner. 2010. 'Corporate Responsibility in Public Health: The Government's Invitation to the Food Industry to Fund Social Marketing on Obesity Is Risky'. *BMJ: British Medical Journal* 341 (7764): 110–11.

MacMillan, T., E. Dowler, and D. Archard. 2006. 'Corporate Responsibility for Children's Diets'. In *Ethics, Law and Society*, edited by J. Gunning and S. Holm, II:237–43. Aldershot: Ashgate.

Marshall, David. 2005. 'Food as Ritual, Routine or Convention'. *Consumption Markets & Culture* 8 (1): 69–85. https://doi.org/10.1080/10253860500069042.

Mol, Annemarie. 2008. *The Logic of Care: Health and the Problem of Patient Choice*. London: Routledge.

Nestle, Marion. 2006. 'Food Industry and Health: Mostly Promises, Little Action'. *The Lancet* 368 (August): 564–65.

———. 2013. *Food Politics : How the Food Industry Influences Nutrition and Health*. Berkeley: University of California Press.

Neve, Kimberley, Corinna Hawkes, Jess Brock, Mark Spires, Charlotte Gallagher Squires, Rosalind Sharpe, Jane Battersby, et al. 2021. 'Understanding Lived Experience of Food Environments to Inform Policy: An Overview of Research Methods'. Centre for Food Policy Research Brief. London: Centre for Food Policy Research.

O'Connell, Rebecca. 2010. '(How) is childminding family like? Family day care, food and the reproduction of identity at the public/private interface.' *The Sociological Review*, 58: 563–86. https://doi.org/10.1111/j.1467-954X.2010.01940.x

O'Connell, Rebecca, and Julia Brannen. 2016. *Food, Families and Work*. London: Bloomsbury.

Overseas Development Institute (ODI). 2015. 'The Price of Vegetables Jumps by up to 91% While the Cost of Some Processed Foods Drops by up to 20%, Driving Obesity – New Report'. *ODI* (blog). 5 May 2015. https://www.odi.org/news/756-price-vegetables-jumps-by-up-91-while-cost-some-processed-foods-drops-by-up-20-driving-obesity-new-report.

Patico, Jennifer, and Eriberto P. Lozada Jr. 2015. 'Children's Food'. In *The Handbook of Food and Anthropology*, edited by Jakob A. Klein and James L. Watson, 200–206. London: Bloomsbury Publishing.

Public Health England, Victoria Targett, and Rachel Allen. 2015. 'Sugar Reduction: The Evidence for Action'. London: Public Health England. https://www.gov.uk/government/uploads/system/uploads/attachment_data/file/470179/Sugar_reduction_The_evidence_for_action.pdf.

Roberts, Kim. 2015. 'Growing Up Not out: The HENRY Approach to Preventing Childhood Obesity'. *British Journal of Obesity* 1 (3): 87–92.

Ulijaszek, Stanley J., and Amy K. McLennan. 2016. 'Framing Obesity in UK Policy from the Blair Years, 1997–2015: The Persistence of Individualistic Approaches despite Overwhelming Evidence of Societal and Economic Factors, and the Need for Collective Responsibility'. *Obesity Reviews* 17 (5): 397–411. https://doi.org/10.1111/obr.12386.

Vallgårda, S., L. Holm, and J. D. Jensen. 2015. 'The Danish Tax on Saturated Fat: Why It Did Not Survive'. *European Journal of Clinical Nutrition* 69 (2): 223–26. https://doi.org/10.1038/ejcn.2014.224.

Wiley, Andrea S. 2011. *Re-Imagining Milk*. New York: Routledge.

———. 2014. 'Milk as a Children's Food: Growth and the Meanings of Milk for Children'. In *Cultures of Milk*, 113–146. Cambridge, MA: Harvard University Press.

3 Feeding children in a childcare setting

Early years settings have historically been developed as sites to encourage specific learning aims and outcomes, as well as more abstract goals related to the shaping of future citizens (Dahlber and Moss 2004, 2). Mealtimes are particularly poignant examples during which this process is at play, and where more intense learning takes place as opposed to allowing activities to be child-led (White 2017), as I witnessed in the year that I spent at Ladybird Nursery and Children's Centre. Several tensions rose between adults and children, but also between staff members, who often had competing views about what needed to be done and achieved when feeding children.

To explore these daily interactions, the chapter first seeks to answer: what are the aims of feeding children in the early years? Based on participant observation and on semi-structured interviews conducted with seven staff members at Ladybird, this chapter will describe the many aspects of feeding children in an early years setting. I will start by looking at how everyday practices within the nursery and children's centre unfolded, how these were shaped by an official discourse that emphasises 'healthy eating,' and how these link to a broader 'civilising process' (Elias 1994; Lupton 1996; Albon and Hellman 2018). Drawing from Flowers and Swan (2016), I argue that to achieve these aims, food and mealtimes were used as 'pedagogical tools' by staff members at Ladybird.

Second, this chapter aims to answer the question: what does feeding children in an early years setting involve? Drawing on Tronto's ethics of care (1993, 2013) framework, as well as wider literature about care and the politics of care work (Abel and Nelson 1990; England and Folbre 1999; Michel 2002; England 2005; Mol 2008), I will describe some of the practical aims that the school staff had to manage during eating events at Ladybird, as well as balancing their personal ethics of care with the logistical aspects of institutional feeding. Drawing from Tronto (1993, 2013) and Abel and Nelson's work on the multifaceted and complex nature of caregiving (1990), I will explain the limits of feeding and caring practices at Ladybird. Further, I will discuss how feeding children in an institutional context also poses some social and emotional limits on early years practitioners, again creating a contrast between their personal ethics of care and the practical aspect of their work.

Finally, my analysis identifies that there is a tension between recognising children's preferences and identities and legitimising the role of the institution

DOI: 10.4324/9781003297642-4

in the eyes of parents and official actors. Ladybird's child-led approach was something that families deemed valuable, yet mealtimes were often far from child-led. Further, following and adhering to official voluntary food and drink guidelines for the early years was necessary for Ladybird to receive a positive outcome in Ofsted reports, however, in the semi-structured interviews it also became apparent that staff members' personal ethics of care did not always match with these aims. The universalism of the bureaucracy, policies, and institutional rules which regulated the daily activities at Ladybird were thus often at odds with the particularism that feeding children in an early years setting requires.

Mealtime schedules

There were four types of mealtimes at Ladybird nursery: breakfast, lunch, snack times, and tea (or supper), and children ate different meals depending on the number of hours they stayed at the nursery.

Breakfast

Breakfast club took place in the children's centre between 8.45 a.m. and 9.20 a.m.; it cost £3 per day, or £2 per day if a family was eligible for free school meals (henceforth, FSM). Breakfast had the fewest amount of children attending, and was the simplest meal of the day; in the months I spent at Ladybird, usually no more than four children came to the sessions, and numbers began dwindling towards the end of the school year, to the point that there were days on which only one family would make use of the service, if at all. Food offered for breakfast included cereal (Weetabix or Rice Krispies),[1] porridge, toast, and milk. Unlike lunch and tea, breakfast was mostly a self-help meal, with children coming in, washing their hands, and helping themselves to what they wanted to drink and eat as they took their seats at the table, where utensils and food were laid out for them. The only food that they needed to request from an adult was toast, which was brought to them from the kitchen.

Lunch

Lunchtime at the nursery took place between 12.00 p.m. and 12.45 p.m., and cost £2 per day unless a child's family was eligible for FSM. This was the occasion that required most preparation and coordination between staff members at Ladybird, as they did not have facilities available to cook lunch on the premises; lunch was thus provided externally by a local catering company. Additional staff support was also needed: the school hired four lunchtime assistants to help at this time, as well as a cook who was responsible for bringing in the food to the classrooms on three trolleys (one for each classroom). As well as lunch, children in the nursery had access to fruit and milk as snacks that they could help themselves to throughout their session (whether they attended nursery full- or part-time).

The school administration aimed to provide a varied lunch menu, which worked on a fortnightly rotation system. Children were offered a main course (which included a vegetarian or a meat-based option), lettuce and other salad vegetables, sliced bread with margarine, a pudding, and fruit. The meat-based options offered were halal for several years, until 2014, when the school administration decided to no longer provide this due to financial constraints. This also had implications on the ways in which staff thought of and addressed dietary diversity and restrictions, as well as how children navigated these differences.

Figures 3.1 and 3.2 show the main courses on two given weeks. Baked potatoes were also provided every day, and although the lunchtime assistants I worked with seemed to view these more as 'backup options' should a child not want to try the main course, it was also common for children to request both a main and a baked potato.

Packed lunches were not permitted at the nursery: families were reassured that all dietary needs and/or allergies would be adequately catered for. Figure 3.3 shows a colour-coded register of children's dietary needs, which lunchtime assistants and teachers consulted during mealtimes – a copy hung in each nursery classroom and at the children's centre. The issue of allergies and dietary requirements was a top priority at Ladybird, as well as across early years settings in the U.K. Providing for any child that might have special dietary needs, and knowing the action plan to follow in case of exposure to allergens, is listed as a requirement that settings should abide by both in the 'Statutory framework for the early years foundation stage' (Department for Education 2017, 28) and Ofsted's 'Early years and child-care registration handbook' (Ofsted 2015, 20), both of which Ladybird followed.

The Children's Trust 'Eat Better Start Better' (EBSB) framework (Children's Food Trust 2012), which I examined in Chapter 1, and to which Ladybird adhered to, also emphasised paying attention to allergies and dietary restrictions, and advised

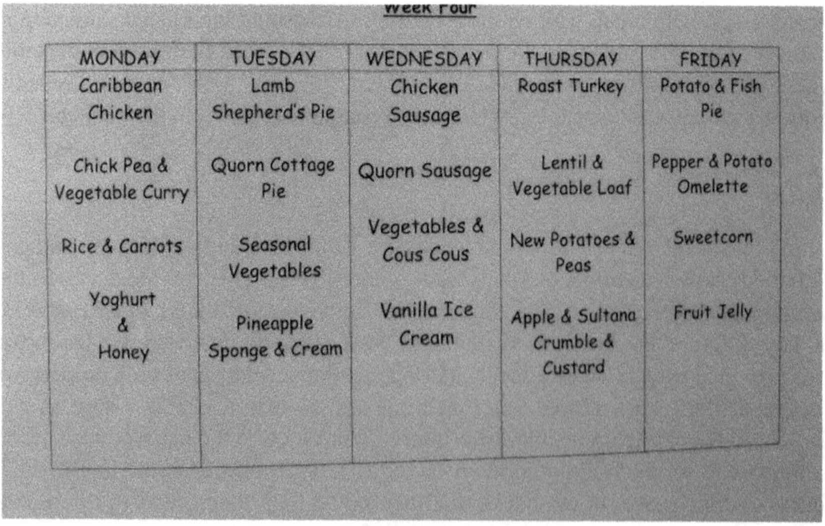

Week Four

MONDAY	TUESDAY	WEDNESDAY	THURSDAY	FRIDAY
Caribbean Chicken	Lamb Shepherd's Pie	Chicken Sausage	Roast Turkey	Potato & Fish Pie
Chick Pea & Vegetable Curry	Quorn Cottage Pie	Quorn Sausage	Lentil & Vegetable Loaf	Pepper & Potato Omelette
Rice & Carrots	Seasonal Vegetables	Vegetables & Cous Cous	New Potatoes & Peas	Sweetcorn
Yoghurt & Honey	Pineapple Sponge & Cream	Vanilla Ice Cream	Apple & Sultana Crumble & Custard	Fruit Jelly

Figure 3.1 Sample lunch menu at Ladybird Nursery, June 2017.

Photograph by the author.

MONDAY	TUESDAY	WEDNESDAY	THURSDAY	FRIDAY
Macaroni Cheese	Chicken Curry	Minced Beef & Vegetable Burritos	Roast Chicken	Breaded Fish Fingers
Peas & Carrots	Sweet Potato & Lentil Curry	Minced Quorn & Vegetable Burritos	Lentil & Vegetable Loaf	Vegetable, Chickpea & Bean Wrap
	Rice & Spinach		Boiled Potatoes & Cauliflower Florets	Oven Chips & Sweetcorn
		Mixed Salad		
Vanilla Ice Cream	Pineapple Crumble & Cream Fraiche	Stewed Pears	Fruit Yoghurt	Sponge & Custard

Figure 3.2 Sample lunch menu at Ladybird Nursery, October 2016.

Photograph by the author.

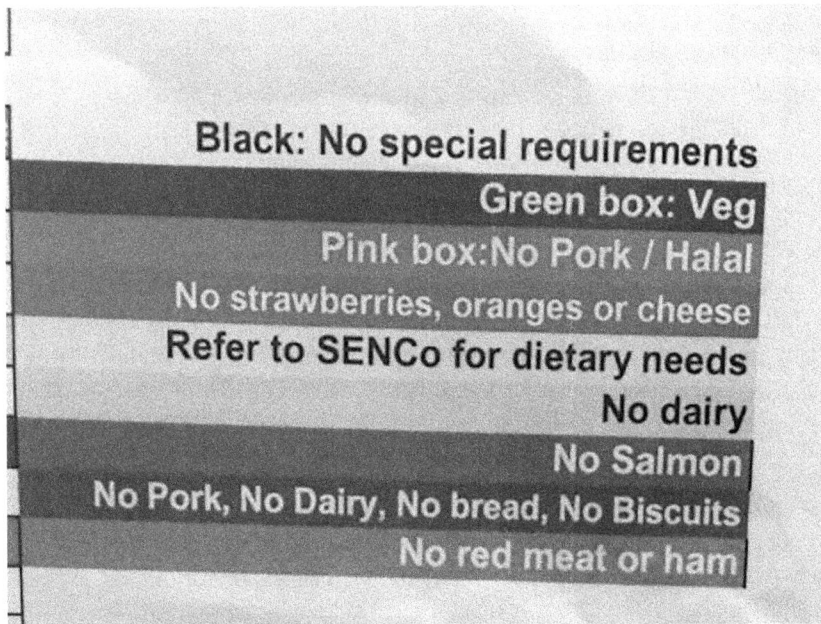

Figure 3.3 A colour-coded register indicating all children's dietary needs. Lunchtime assistants consulted this guide during mealtimes.

Photograph by the author.

settings to 'develop allergy plans' (ibid., 15) to offset the dangers associated to allergic reactions. Much has been written on how the rise of a 'risk society' (Beck 1992) has had an evident impact on parents' (particularly mothers') feeding practices (see, e.g. Murphy 2000; Afflerback et al. 2013; Faircloth 2014), and this certainly extends into institutional settings. An increased emphasis on risk, paired to audit culture, has meant that all foods (not just allergens or contaminated food, but also foods that could be a choking hazard) are often perceived as a source of potential danger.

At 11.45 a.m., after time spent playing outdoors, two children from each classroom were asked to help set the tables in preparation for lunchtime, which involved placing cutlery and a plastic cup in front of each seat. Lunch assistants would lay out the cups and cutlery for them to place in front of each seat. The rest of the children were then called inside from the playground and ushered towards the toilets and asked to wash their hands before they took their seats – usually they were free to choose their own places, unless the teachers or lunchtime assistants thought that a given group dynamic would "cause trouble." After everyone was seated, Mary, the cook, brought in the lunch trolleys, and the food was served one by one to the children by the lunchtime assistants, who sat with the children and ate with them. Every child was made to "scrape" the leftovers off their plates into a nearby plastic bowl after they finished eating their main meal and dessert.

'Tea-club' (snack and supper)

Some children with working parents also stayed for 'tea-club,' which took place between 3.15 p.m. and 5.45 p.m. Two meals were offered at tea-club; first, a snack consisting of fruit and "a portion of carbohydrates" (as it was called in the 'Eat Better Start Better' guidelines, which were followed to prepare the food at tea-club),[2] together with milk and water. Some children were be picked up shortly after this snack, at 4.20 p.m.; the remaining 'tea-clubbers' were served supper at this point. The tea-club fee if the child only stayed for the snack was £3 per day (or £2 per day if the family was eligible for FSM), or £7 if the child also stayed for supper (or £4 if the family was eligible for FSM). Although a menu (similar to the lunch menu) was also issued for tea-club, during the year that I spent at Ladybird it was not necessarily the case that staff members in charge of running the sessions would follow this. If the ingredients needed to make that day's meal suggestion were available then the menu would be followed, yet the children would more often be offered whatever was available in the fridge/freezer and cupboard, which did not always correspond to the menu. Typical meals served for supper would be pasta with pesto or tomato sauce, rice with vegetables, or fish fingers and peas. Towards the end of the school year that I spent at Ladybird, the school's administration decided that lunch leftovers should be served at tea-club to avoid food waste. However, this meant that some children ate the same meal twice on the same day.

Other mealtimes

Food was also offered to the infants who attended activities at the children's centre, at no extra cost for the parents. A snack consisting of fruit and "a portion of carbohydrates" was given at the end of every 'stay-and-play' session, which was eaten communally. At this time especially, parents were encouraged to interact with their children by sitting with them and by helping the staff serve the food and drinks. Fruit and a carbohydrate-based snack were also given to children who stayed at the crèche, available to parents who attended English, maths, or other lessons in the adjoining training room; crèche was the only childcare service at Ladybird in which parents were allowed to provide packed food for their children.

Exploring the aims of feeding children in the early years

Food as a pedagogical tool

Drawing from Flowers and Swan (2016), I conceptualise food as a pedagogical tool following their definition of 'food pedagogies,' a term they coined to make sense of the rise in education initiatives about food and diet, together with the appearance of new communities of experts that communicate knowledge and information about food (2016, 22). These authors further contend that there is a multiplicity of contexts within which food pedagogies are operationalised (ibid.), with schools being of particular interest as a site where food and eating are closer to the culture of risk already mentioned (ibid., 32). At Ladybird, this way of thinking about food – as a pedagogical tool and to be managed as a risk – played an important role structuring mealtimes, and the aims and task(s) of providing food to children.

The concept of the 'pedagogical meal,' which originates in Sweden (Gullberg 2006; Benn and Carlsson 2014), entails the use of food as a means of learning about the wider world. Benn and Carlsson suggest that a 'pedagogical meal' encourages children and childcare workers to spend time together, as well as being a time for learning and expressing care (2014, 24). My observations of mealtimes at Ladybird revealed that food could be used pedagogically in a narrower way: first, in how it was used to teach children about 'healthy eating' and, second, in how it was central in promoting 'table manners,' which relates to the idea of the 'civilised body' or 'civilised self' discussed in Chapter 1. The way in which eating and table manners are implicated in the 'civilising process' – which children are meant to be engaged in from a young age – was famously first interrogated by Elias in *The Civilizing Process* (1994). Elias argues that social rules and expectations have a huge impact on children, even from a young age, so that they are faced with the options of either accepting the norms imposed on them by society or to be otherwise excluded from it (1994, 116).

Whilst Elias' work has been greatly influential in food and childhood studies, it also has its limitations. In line with other childhood scholars, Albon and Hellman contend that children are social agents who actively participate and influence their social worlds, rather than being passive learners (2018, 13), a vision which is absent in Elias' work. Van Krieken has argued that Elias thought of the process of civilisation as one that relies on a constantly evolving 'psychic structure' which shapes social relationships and 'instinctual life' (1998, 90–91). This also poses some limitations on the way children and childhood are currently construed in childhood studies, as well as in this book: children are viewed as actively engaged with the social worlds around them and partaking in dialogic (Bakhtin 1986) relations with their peers and adults. What should nonetheless be noted is the influence of Elias' work on poststructuralist scholarship, which pays attention to how knowledge and discourse has been shaped historically. For example, Lupton contends that norms and values around food and eating epitomise the idea of a 'civilised body' that surveils itself and other bodies (1996, 22). Similarly, Fischler argues that eating shapes social and individual behaviours on both social (macro) and biological (micro) dimensions (2011, 534).

At Ladybird, food and meals were used as pedagogical tools in a number of ways: to teach children about 'healthy eating,' to teach them about table manners, and to overcome 'fussy eating.' The EBSB programme, which I examined in Chapter 1, also emphasises that "learning about and through food can be linked to the Early Years Foundation Stage (EYFS) curriculum" (Children's Food Trust 2012, 53). Further, a whole section of the handbook is dedicated to help practitioners to "Encourag[e] fussy eaters to eat well" (ibid., 51). This highlights once again the interplay between education policy and public health in the discourse about children's food.

Conceptualising food as a pedagogical tool is useful to understand the rationale that guided and shaped the aims and practices of many of the staff members that worked at Ladybird. This came across in an interview with Sima, one of four lunchtime assistants that worked at Ladybird. She was born in England from Indian parents and had been working at Ladybird for nine years at the time of our interview:

FV: *So what do you think is the most important part of your job as a lunchtime assistant?*

SIMA: *To make sure that the children have a nutritional, balanced diet during lunch, and encouraging the child to try different foods. Because certain children are just used [...] to their traditional foods...it's really important that we open them up to all the different kinds of food that [...] is available...and encourage them to try, you know, a little bit. Just licking it or even having it on their plate is an achievement for some of them. Because [with] some of them it's just a complete, "No"...and if some of them get too emotional about it, if it's too stressful, you know, each child is different so you have to go with each child, you can't just have the same...how can I put it...routine for all of them, like, "OK, we're going to give you everything on your plate, all you children have the same," because it doesn't work, as you've seen, some children get too emotional when they don't want something on their plate. And just that they enjoy it [lunchtime] as well. Eating can be fun as well. So letting them experiment, even if it means touching and feeling as well, it's important...yeah, we encourage them to use their knives and forks but it's important to have the sensory...because there are children...like, in my tradition [Indian], we use our hands to eat, so a lot of children that do come, we tend to notice that they really do use their fingers and their hands to eat, because that's what they're used to back home. So yeah, just understanding every child's background, because we have such diverse children that come in, it's important to understand what their background is as well.*

Sima'sresponse to a question I asked all staff, What do you think is the most important aspect of your job?, is emblematic of the topics this chapter seeks to explore because, in a couple of minutes, she referred to most of the things that needed to be taken into consideration – almost simultaneously – by the staff members who provided food to children at Ladybird. Her account touches upon the matter of healthy eating, promoting 'good manners,' encouraging children to "try a bit of everything," being attuned to the 'routine' of each child, as she put it, as well as the children's diverse ethnic and cultural backgrounds, and how these might shape their food preferences.

Having paid attention to Sima's practices at lunchtime, the response she gave to my question made sense. One day she asked me to help her by sitting at her table, because Amir (four), who was perceived by staff members to be one of the children that needed more attention, was sitting with her. One of the points she expressed to me in the interview, that "*each child is different so you have to go with each child,*" was put into practice that day, both to "*keep Amir calm,*" as she would later tell me, as well as to encourage Karolina (also four) to eat vegetables. On this particular day, a Friday, fish and chips was on the menu. In my fieldnotes I noted:

Karolina says she only wants fish (no chips or veggies), so Sima makes an 'animal' on her plate to encourage her to eat more than just fish. The fish is the 'body,' the chips are the 'legs,' a piece of cucumber is the 'head,' and a bit of lettuce is the 'grass' (which Karolina especially doesn't want). She eats the fish heartily, some of the chips and cucumbers, but leaves the piece of lettuce aside, showing her disgust for it when Sima asks her if she's going to try it – fieldnotes, February 2017.

Indeed, throughout my time at Ladybird, I noticed Sima using the strategy of creating images with the food, as described above. This is something we also talked about during the interview:

FV: *I've noticed you have very creative strategies to encourage the children to eat...*

SIMA: *Yes, the smiley faces! Yeah, especially with the fruit, that helps them, because it encourages them, they find it fun, they don't realise that they're actually eating a fruit, when one is picking the nose and it's a banana, or an orange, or pear, or whatever it is we've got on the plate...they're a bit hesitant to try, but I've started noticing that [it works] when I put it in a funny face.*

Her attitude towards Amir also seemed equally thought through. In my fieldnotes I noted:

> *After he is done eating, Amir starts to get restless: he leaves his chair and starts walking around the classroom. Instead of telling him to sit down again (as other lunchtime assistants or teachers often, impatiently, tend to do), Sima asks him to help her by taking different bits of crockery to the lunch trolley while the other children finish their lunch. She does this little by little, giving him one thing at the time so that the process lasts until lunch is over. She gives him the fish tray last, because she knew he was going to take a piece out of the tray to eat – this amuses both Sima and Amir. She turns to me and says, "I knew he was going to do that!" and then to him, "I told Fran, I knew you were going to do that!", and the three of us laugh [...] Afterwards, in the playground, Sima tells me it's important to know the different ways to "deal with the challenges" that come up at lunchtime, recounting the "strategies" she used with Karolina and Amir earlier: "You just need to keep him [Amir] occupied," she tells me. About Karolina she says, "You need to be creative to get them to eat. You learn these things over time" – fieldnotes, February 2017.*

The attention Sima afforded to her role as lunchtime assistant was not necessarily unique, yet she articulated the link between her thoughts and actions a lot more explicitly than some of the other lunchtime assistants. This is in line with Tronto's definition of care as practice, involving "both thought and action" (1993, 108). Sima's account also reveals something important about the intentions most staff members shared if their role was (or included) providing food to the children: indeed, 'getting' children to try 'a bit of everything' was perceived as crucial by most staff, and something that many parents also expected the school to help with (as also outlined in the EYFS or EBSB frameworks). The tension between the universalism of bureaucracy and policy, and the particularism that feeding children in childcare necessitates is also brought to evidence by Sima's reflections and practices: as Mol argues, 'good care' demands that attention be paid to detail (2008, 67). Sima seemed to be able to balance these two dimensions of her job, yet it was not the case that all staff members were able to do the same.

Sima's practices, nonetheless, also reveal some contradictions. In her account, she emphasised making mealtimes a pleasurable and enjoyable experience for the children, but ultimately the pedagogical outcomes of the meal seemed to take precedence. For instance, making food arrangements on children's plates to encourage them to eat shows that adults can mirror children's behaviours to help them pursue their own goals. Writing about marketing of food to children, Elliott coins the term 'eatertainment' (2010) to explain how the food industry has incorporated the ideas of 'fun' and 'play' to advertise food products to children.[3] Whilst playing with one's food was not generally encouraged or sanctioned by the staff at Ladybird, Sima's approach can be categorised as 'eatertainment.' It shows that certain rules could be bent if this served a wider pedagogical purpose, like encouraging 'fussy eaters' to 'try a bit of everything.'

The 'problem' of 'fussy eating'

Four-year-old Karolina was one of the children whose family had concerns about her 'fussy eating,' and thus who the staff were paying particular attention to during all the mealtimes that she partook in at Ladybird. In my fieldnotes, I wrote about Karolina's first day attending breakfast club:

> *Today is the first day that Karolina joins breakfast club. When Karolina and her mother arrive, Ruby [in charge of breakfast and tea-club] introduces herself to Karolina, and tells her that she'll be the person that she will see in the mornings. While Karolina joins me and the other two children at the table, Olga, Karolina's mother, explains to Ruby that Robert [extended services manager] recommended that she bring Karolina to breakfast club for a trial period, because she is having trouble getting her to wake up in the mornings and to eat something before coming to school. After Olga leaves, Ruby asks Karolina what she'd like for breakfast, listing all the options (Weetabix, porridge, Rice Krispies, and toast) and Karolina chooses toast. While the bread is toasting Ruby also asks Karolina what she would like to drink (milk or water) and Karolina refuses both, shaking her head. Once the toast is ready, Ruby joins us at the table, asking Karolina what she would like on her bread (margarine or jam, or both) and Karolina points at the margarine. Ruby helps Karolina spread it on her toast by holding her hand with the knife. Karolina eats all of it promptly, just leaving the crusts on her plate [...] Later, while Ruby and I clean up after the children have gone to nursery, she and Robert assess Karolina's first session at breakfast club. He asks Ruby what Karolina ate, and Ruby says she wanted toast with margarine. Robert says that fussy eaters should initially be given what they ask for, "because this is important if we're trying to get fussy children to eat." He adds that he thinks Karolina was weaned only on purees, which is an issue, because when 'normal' food is presented to children weaned on mainly purees they find it strange: "They see broccoli and they're like, why did you put a tree on my plate?!" he says. He tells Ruby that the "way forward" with Karolina is to give her lots of "encouragement and praise" during mealtimes – fieldnotes, December 2016.*

Ruby's and Robert's approach with Karolina echoes the idea that early years settings have increasingly adopted a range of mechanisms and techniques to create "a particular subject [...] the autonomous and flexible child" (Dahlberg and Moss 2004, 2). Ruby's encouragement to make Karolina choose the food she wants to eat and helping her to butter her toast by placing the knife in her hand is linked to the notion of autonomy that Dahlberg and Moss allude to. The ability to make the 'right choices' in relation to food also reflects the official discourses about food and eating that I explored in Chapter 1; whilst in the example above Robert emphasises that initially Karolina should be praised for eating anything she likes, the ultimate goal is for Karolina to be able to make 'healthy choices' in the future, and to be flexible enough to try a variety of foods.

The aim of 'getting' children to try different things, or to overcome their 'fussiness,' is one example of the ways in which power relations between children and adults unfolded at Ladybird. It also makes evident that a tension exists between acknowledging children's preferences and validating the institution, which some staff members seemed to recognise. Joyce, the lead early years practitioner at the children's centre, said:

> *It's what **they** [the adults] want them [the children] to eat, not what the kids want. It's not what they try, it doesn't matter, as long as they eat this much of that [...] If the kid is being fussy and all they want is potato, I'm like, well yeah, let them have it. Obviously they should be encouraged to try everything but here [in the UK] they're like, 'Well if they don't want that just let them go hungry for a bit,' but I'm not comfortable with that. No parent ever is. And I would never...I would never be one to suggest that. I don't agree with that, and I just can't keep my professional hat on, so if parents ask me what to do because their kid is only eating potato I tell them, let them eat it, at least they're eating. And it's not like they're going to do it until they're 25, kids go through phases – semi-structured interview, July 2017.*

Joyce's account shows that when there were discrepancies between staff's rationales and aims, the possibility to enter or empathise with children's viewpoints also existed, limiting the extent to which adults felt it was necessary to always embody a disciplining role. Joyce's statement also challenges some of the official narrative on the irreversibility of what children experience in the early years, pointing out that "*kids go through phases.*"

Staff's commitment to encourage 'fussy eaters' to try different things thus varied. Some, like Joyce, believed that if children were eating at all this was a good thing, others were more committed to encouraging children try different foods. Cynthia, one of the nursery teachers who sometimes helped during lunchtime, was more persistent about this. When she served lunch to the children she would tell them they had to choose at least one vegetable, and if they refused she would pick one for them herself, saying, "*Try **just** a little bit.*" She also used alliteration when offering food to them, asking "*Who would like some lovely lettuce?*" or "*crunchy carrot,*" for instance, phrases that the children would often echo to each other during other mealtimes, such as tea-club. Her attempts were not always successful, however, and they often resisted these invitations to try something new:

> *For dessert today there is vanilla sponge cake and single cream to pour on top. Cynthia asks each child around the table if they would like cream on their cake when she passes the plate to them, and none of them do. When she gives the cake to Amir she asks him, "Amir **are you sure** you don't want to try some [cream]?" and Linda [four] humorously but assertively interjects before he can answer: "**No one** wants to try some Cynthia!" – fieldnotes, January 2017.*

'Fussy eaters' were thus very much seen as in need of adults' intervention to correct their behaviour. From a medical anthropological standpoint, 'fussy eating' can be understood as a way in which behaviours that are seen as out of the norm can be framed as problematic and further validated as such by the biomedical sphere. Although 'fussy eating' cannot really be compared to a medical diagnosis, it is a concern that many parents asked the school's advice on, and for which some also sought medical help, as I observed during the sessions with the dietician at Ladybird. Considering that most children might at one point or another be called 'fussy,' and in light of the fact that, as Lupton contends, children can often assert their agency by refusing food or eating 'bad' foods (1996, 55–56), it seems pertinent to question what the aim of labelling a child 'fussy' is. Indeed, this calls to mind ongoing debates on ADHD diagnoses for children, for example, which some have described as "the medicalization of what is essentially normal child behaviour" (Wiley and Allen 2013, 258; see also Rafalovich 2013). The term 'fussy eater' also links to a particular vision of the child as malleable, and as simultaneously in need of protection but also intervention (Moran-Ellis 2010, 189, 197). At Ladybird, whilst there were times (particularly tea-club) in which staff viewed children as more independent, and during which more attention was paid to what they deemed meaningful about mealtimes, 'fussy eaters' were very much seen as in need of adults' intervention to correct their behaviour.

'Healthy eating' in the early years

Addressing the issue of 'fussy eating' was also closely linked to promoting 'healthy eating habits,' since the foods children were often reluctant to try were 'healthy foods,' such as vegetables. Ruby was the staff member who was most involved in talking to children about 'healthy eating' (as she was also leading the EBSB initiative at the children's centre). Since she began working at Ladybird in November 2016, Ruby spoke about healthy eating to the children who attended breakfast or tea-club practically every day. In our interview, she linked her commitment to talking about healthy eating with her concern about the rise in childhood obesity. She also echoed notions about the importance of early intervention and the idea that by making more information available health behaviours will improve, both of which are still prevalent in current education and public health discourse. During our interview, I asked her whether talking to children about healthy eating was something she had done throughout her career:

RUBY: *In my other school I worked with reception children [four- to five-year-olds] and we would have a snack time. At about half past ten, we would all sit on the carpet and it would just be me and the children. And they would have their snack, and it would be fruit and milk. So it's the perfect opportunity to talk about healthy eating, talk to them about the milk...because children, sometimes they don't know where the milk comes from. They think it comes from the shop. Because I did ask some children, recently, about food, and they said it's from the shop, so they don't actually know that some foods...that the milk comes from the cow, and the cow lives in the farm. So...you know, it's just giving them information [...] Because there is so much information out there about healthy eating, I don't think*

> *we should have obese children [...] The amount of information, technol-*
> *ogy that we've got out there...we shouldn't have it.*
>
> FV: *And do you think the early years is the right time to start [talking about*
> *healthy eating]?*
>
> RUBY: *Yes. I mean, they know it, and I have said to them, that you will need to*
> *know this...if you want to be healthy [...] all these things I'm telling you,*
> *you will need to know when you're a grown up because it will help you to*
> *stay healthy. And they know if you don't eat healthy food you will get sick,*
> *you will get fat so...they understand the benefits of it, so I hope...I know*
> *for reception, anyway, it will be encouraged [and] when they go on to*
> *other years, that they will still encourage it.*

The children's centre, with its involvement in the EBSB campaign, and being part of the Mixed Economy of Welfare (MEW) (Powell 2014), was where children and families were most exposed to "public health imperatives" (Leahy and Malins 2015) about nutrition. Ruby echoed the concern for childhood obesity and high sugar intake prevalent in official discourses about children's food. The notions of 'choice,' and that information and knowledge about 'healthy eating' are key determinants of health outcomes, were also central to our conversation – notions that tend to underplay the material constraints that have an impact on people's diets. Ruby's personal ethics of care seemed to be tied to the biomedical and policy discourses about children's food.

Similarly, in the interview I conducted with Robert, he expressed that, as manager of the children's centre, he was invested in bringing some of his personal values about 'healthy' food and eating to the setting:

> *I felt really strongly [that] coming into this role was about educating families,*
> *and trying to improve health outcomes. So there are a number of priorities*
> *the local authority asked me to look at, health being one of them [...] So*
> *my interest in healthy eating, personally, I wanted to operate professionally*
> *[...] I was shocked that there was very little information or guidance other*
> *than, look, here are the stats. So you were seeing the data but there was no*
> *real drive or initiative to it [...] I thought that I would like our community to*
> *have a setting where that becomes a bigger focus over a period of time [...]*
> *So that's what I did. So the first part was about any of the provision where*
> *we incorporate a snack we took out the toast and we had milk, water [...]*
> *And no juice, no cordial...and I incorporated fruit into the snack times. So*
> *there was a bread stick and then a choice of fruit, and that's what it became.*
> *So I removed the toast, and actually did that across the nursery and here*
> *[the children's centre] [...] So that was the first bit. For the extended day, so*
> *that's breakfast and tea club, we were offering toast in the mornings and Rice*
> *Krispies, I think. And then in the evening we had [laughs] like chips, chicken*
> *nuggets, the usual, frozen commodity stuff, and tins. So that was the next part*
> *to really try and tackle, which is still evolving, we're not there yet [...] So*
> *the main part was trying to come away from prepared, processed foods to a*
> *more fresh-food based approach – semi-structured interview, August 2017.*

Robert's account here also echoes Public Health England and NHS nutrition-driven discourses about healthy eating, which prioritises freshly made food, fruits, and vegetables over processed foods. Removing juice and cordial from the setting addresses ongoing concerns with children's sugar consumption, which were indeed prevalent among the staff at Ladybird, as well as parents. Robert's ambition to "educate families" and "improve health outcomes," as a response to some of the aims the local government was seeking to achieve, is also an example of how MEW functions in practice. As Powell puts forward, within the MEW model "well-being does not depend solely on politicians, but also on individuals acting as purchasers or carers, voluntary organisations and employers. In many ways, people make their own social policies, but not in circumstances of their choosing" (2014, 236). That Robert felt that he should put the task of improving the food standards at Ladybird, and give information to parents, into his own hands, with few resources available, reflects Powell's argument that "people make their own social policies" (ibid.), but also the issues that arise when the welfare state shrinks and health is predominantly linked to individual accountability.

Robert's remarks also highlight the contrasts between what children and adults might deem valuable about school food. As Hansen and Kristensen have pointed out for the Danish childcare context, feeding children is a rational, long-term project where food is perceived as 'fuel,' and care is (among other things) a health promotion endeavour (2017, 494). Yet, perhaps most importantly, the link made between promoting 'healthy eating' within the setting and that of "educating families" suggests that the use of food as a pedagogical tool is not limited to the school, but often extends into the home environment. Since Donzelot's seminal work *The Policing of Families* (1977), ample literature has emerged suggesting that schools in advanced liberal societies have become sites in which governmental techniques (Foucault 1991) are enacted. Schools can target and seek to improve parental behaviour following various public health discourses (e.g. Crozier 1998; Baez and Talburt 2008; Maher, Fraser, and Wright 2010; Pike and Leahy 2012).[4]

Table manners, school readiness, and perceptions of the home environment

In the English ECEC policy context, growing attention is being placed on school readiness and other future outcomes, versus valuing children's experiences in the present. Mealtimes at Ladybird showed many examples of how this can manifest in practice. For Ruby and Robert, eating 'healthy,' learning table manners, and school readiness were deeply interrelated. In our interview, Ruby said:

> *The transition from nursery to reception is very different [to transitions within nursery], because the children in the reception age group eat in a big hall...and it's very, it's big, there's rows...the comfy environment that you have in nursery, it's not like that in the schools. So children could get lost in that kind of setting, so it would be good if they had the social skills to be able to still be able to sit and talk to each other about food, talk about their day [...] there's things they would never talk about, but when they're sitting*

down eating they're comfortable, so they will express themselves, they will say things which they might not normally say – semi-structured interview, July 2017.

Ruby encouraged this kind of interaction both at breakfast and tea-club, although predominantly during the latter, when there was more time and more children were present. If children communicated nonverbally, by nodding or pointing, for instance, she asked them to "*use their words*" to say what they wanted. She reminded them to say "please" and "thank you" and often would not respond to children's requests if they did not say these words. If children asked for help with a task that Ruby considered feasible for them to do on their own (such as pouring themselves a drink), she would refuse and say that they needed to learn "*how to be independent, which means doing things for yourself*," emphasising that this would be expected of them in "big school" (as she and others referred to primary school).

Similarly, when Robert and I discussed the consequences that the 30-hours free childcare allowance for working parents[5] would have on the number of children having meals at Ladybird nursery, he said:

So the impact I believe [...] is that there will be less opportunities for children to eat together, to have those really enriching experiences, those children that will be accessing food will be those with parents that are working, that are probably already coming from backgrounds where...they're not strangers to sitting down having a healthy meal. That's quite...it sounds quite judgemental, and I don't mean it in that way, but what we tend to see is that those families that are in working households tend to have less vulnerabilities, there is more structure to their life, they, not always, but tend to sit together and eat together...as opposed to those that come from different situations – semi-structured interview, August 2017.

The idea that much of ECEC policy exists to address perceived shortcomings or deficiencies in the home environment is clear in the available literature (e.g. Clarke 2006; Camps and Long 2012; Moss 2012; Sayer 2017). Staff's perceptions of parents, and children's home environments, is an important final point to address in answering the question about the aims of feeding children in the early years, as well as their perceptions about the link between poverty and diet, which could be contradictory at times. In the interview I conducted with Fatima, one of the lunchtime assistants, she told me:

I think that we are in the generation of wealth. In the past, I think poverty was more so, when people were rationing their food at home. And so, we are exposed to so much choice that I think you can still be healthy if you don't have so much money, and make the right choices with food, because I do believe we are in a generation that is wealthy and a lot of choices are out there, it's just about making the right choices – semi-structured interview, July 2017.

In line with the notion that individual behaviour is a key determinant of health outcomes, some staff, like Fatima, individualised responsibility for food and eating and minimised the role of material constraints, by focusing on the idea of personal 'choice' that is advanced in nutrition-driven discourses about food and eating. As shown above, Ruby had similar views. During our interview, she added:

> *I was brought up in a poor family. I am the seventh child of eight. And you can still have healthy food. You just need to know what food to buy [...] I don't have loads of money, I don't want to spend lots of money on food anyway...if you've got [...] good value for money food, I'm going to buy it [...] The government do help people on low incomes, they get vouchers, they get food vouchers, it's just how...what choices you're making with that...so, really I think it is education.*

Another lunchtime assistant, Joanne, echoed these notions about choice, whilst simultaneously drawing from personal experience to assess whether it is possible to make 'good choices' when faced with financial hardship:

JOANNE: *I also think it's about how you cook...I think as well, making good choices, with parents who're cooking...you know, with the oils and that kind of stuff...*

FV: *Some of the parents have told me they often don't have enough time to think too much about what they're going to cook...*

JOANNE: *It's preparation really. It's about preparing yourself. And sometimes if you haven't got the money or the time, it's difficult. I find with myself, if I know what I'm going to eat for the next few days...you can organise it more. But if you're just sort of like...if some people haven't got the money, they just make do with what they've got...you know, so it is very difficult [...] Because you've got to have that money to have that stuff indoors, you know. And it's quite easy to go to the freezer and get some chips and some nuggets out of the freezer. I mean I've never bought nuggets...because I don't agree with that, but that's me. But I've had to do when I didn't have money. It's just making good choices. I mean, you can buy vegetables, but some things are quite expensive now...I mean I have turned that around because life has gotten a lot easier for me as I've got older...but I was widowed with two babies so young...I was on benefits trying to get to make ends meet...you can't always do it. So I've been there, so I sort of know, you know? It was difficult.*

In Chapter 1, I explored how the role of material constraints is minimised in policy by focusing on the idea of personal 'choice' in official discourse. These accounts, in turn, shed light on how seemingly contradictory narratives (that making 'good' choices is easy, but that 'healthy' food is expensive, for instance) can similarly become intertwined in mainstream discourse when responsibility for food and eating is individualised.

The link between income, parenting, and eating practices will be discussed at length in Chapter 5. However, in initially looking at these accounts, it is relevant to note staff's belief that mealtimes at Ladybird, with their overarching aim to overcome 'fussiness,' and to promote 'healthy eating,' 'good manners,' and school readiness, were particularly important for children coming from less affluent backgrounds. On the one hand, this reflected concerns about some children's lack of access to nutritious food; for example, during the first few months of my fieldwork, Joyce told me that she knew that the fruit provided at the children's centre might be the only fruit some of the children had during the week. On the other hand, this also seemed to mirror an assumption that mealtimes are fundamental to introduce children to the norms of 'civilised' behaviour (Lupton 1996, 38), and there seemed to be an implicit aim to compensate at school for perceived deficiencies within some of the children's homes. In the ECEC context within which Ladybird exists, not only are children being engaged in a 'civilising process' (Elias 1994; Lupton 1996, 22), but, in several cases, so are the parents.

Having explored the different aims early years practitioners pursued when feeding children, by using food and mealtimes as pedagogical tools, the following section will discuss some of the practicalities, situations, and relationships that the staff had to manage daily, which went beyond providing food, but which happened in relation to it.

"His mummy is coming because he's been sick": mealtimes and the ethics of care

Fieldnotes, November 2016:

Things are going relatively smoothly during lunchtime today, until Timur [four] starts coughing. When it stops he starts forcing himself to cough again. He tells Cynthia, "I'm coughing!", bringing his situation to her attention, and Cynthia says, reassuringly, "Yes, and you were a bit sick last week, but you're OK today." Timur pulls his t-shirt up saying, "Mummy opened my tummy," and Cynthia replies, "Yes, she lifted your top to check your belly because you were sick, but you're OK today." Despite Cynthia's attempts to reassure Timur, he keeps making himself cough and starts saying, "I need to go to the toilet." Cynthia continues trying to calm him down; he keeps coughing and starts making throwing up sounds – eventually he persuades Cynthia to let him go to the toilet [adjacent to the tables where lunch is served] and we hear him coughing more. She turns to me and says, with resignation, "Ah and now he's gone to make himself sick in the toilet," and gets up to assist him.

Fieldnotes, December 2016:

[During lunch] Timur coughs until he starts being sick. He throws up a bit in his mouth, which he covers, and then Fatima urges him to go to the toilet, speaking to him in Turkish. She goes with him to the toilet and comes out shortly after to call Timur's mum. We can still hear Timur being sick in the bathroom.

Vomiting was a common, yet disruptive, occurrence at Ladybird, and one that encapsulates several of the dynamics that this chapter seeks to unpack. Vomiting directly interfered with attempts to regulate children's eating, but required an extra level of attention and care from the staff. As Abel and Nelson contend, bureaucratic practices and professionalism within institutions distance carers from those receiving care (1990, 13), so that caregivers' personal experiences and knowledge(s) are devalued in the caregiving encounter. The very mechanisms that are in place to ensure care can also produce certain limitations when they interact with the contingencies and practical constraints that arise within institutions in day-to-day interactions.

As shown in the accounts and practices of the Ladybird staff, this balancing between bureaucratic processes and personal ethics of care could be challenging. Some of the staff, like Sima, were able to implement their own views in their practice with ease while others felt much more constrained by the logistical dimension that their work entailed. In the context of feeding children, particularly in the early years, this dynamic between institutional rules and the emotional/intrapersonal aspect of caregiving is additionally complicated, because of the associations of closeness and nurture inherent in the act of feeding (e.g. Emond, McIntosh, and Punch 2014; Hansen and Kristensen 2017) and the still widely held assumption that childcare provision acts as a replacement for parental (specifically motherly) care (e.g. Moss and Petrie 2000; Brooker 2010).

The limits of carework, particularly childcare, can be especially blurry and emotionally charged as shown, for example, by Emond et al. in an ethnographic account of feeding practices in residential childcare homes in Scotland (Emond, McIntosh, and Punch 2014). Here, the authors found that "professional rules could restrict the extent to which children were allowed to be cared for before staff actions and feelings were perceived as 'unprofessional'" (ibid., 1850). Similarly, when children vomited at Ladybird some of the contradictions that carework entails were revealed. On the one hand, a child that was unwell required closer attention and care from the staff, whilst simultaneously they were distanced though several bureaucratic procedures which, ultimately, resulted in parents taking their child home. Getting children to go home was not necessarily only related to staff's concern for the well-being of the child that got sick, or fear that other children might also become ill. Surprisingly to me, there was a general consensus among the staff that children deliberately made themselves sick because they 'knew' that their parents would come to pick them up.

For example, one day, Jade, one of the girls that stayed at the weekly crèche,[6] was intensely sick for a third time over the span of just a few weeks. After the event, I expressed my concern to Joyce about the fact that I had observed some of the children, like Timur and Jade, regularly being sick:

Joyce says that it's probably nothing to worry about. She tells me small children's stomachs are more sensitive to stimuli and that crying [Jade had been crying intensely before being sick] makes their stomachs move in a "contracting way" that leads to vomiting – she compares it to the procedure of pumping someone's stomach, saying that the movements provoked in people whose stomachs are being pumped are similar to those of children when they cry. She also says that vomiting is a "form of control," and a way of "getting their mummies" as children "know" that we will call them if they are ill – fieldnotes, October 2016.

Perhaps it was indeed the case that children were well aware of the effects of being sick at school. On another occasion, when Oscar (four) vomited on the table during lunchtime and one of the teachers left the room to use the phone, the children discussed this in agreement with each other: "*They're calling his mummy because he's been sick.*"

As well as disrupting the daily routine, vomiting is also an extreme example of the many practical and logistical aspects that carework (and feeding children) entail in an institutional context. In my fieldnotes from October, I wrote about the system in place to clean up vomit:

The procedure in place to clean/sanitise the room after this kind of incident happens involves lots of tissue to initially soak up the fluid, disposable gloves (to pick up the tissues and wipe the area), a powder sanitizer that gets sprinkled over the vomit (this dries up the liquid, making into a powder which then gets vacuumed) and a designated 'sick bucket' that Mark [the janitor] brings in to mop the floor with after this kind of incident (we also have a green plastic brush and dustpan labelled 'SICK' that we use to collect any leftover waste after vacuuming). Joyce collects any toys that were in the area in which Jade vomited, and soaks them in the kitchen sink with liquid sanitizer. My soiled clothes are collected by Joanne and taken to be washed and dried in the nursery's laundry facilities. While we wait for Jade's mother to collect her, we leave Jade sitting on the little couch in the kitchen corner to recover. As on other occasions when children have been sick, we tell other children not to approach the person who has just vomited: both staff and children give the child who has been sick some "quiet time" until their parent arrives to collect them – fieldnotes, October 2016.

In the time I spent doing fieldwork, there were no alternatives to the procedure I have described above, and all the staff seemed to agree that there was little cause for concern if a child vomited because they generally did so intentionally. Nonetheless, these rules also posed restrictions on how a child could be comforted in that situation. Similarly to the study by Emond et al. quoted above (2014), in which displaying emotions or feelings to children in residential care might have been considered 'unprofessional,' deviating from these rules would have been deemed inappropriate by some staff at Ladybird, yet not everyone thought it was best to isolate the child while they waited to be picked up, or that they needed "quiet time." The rules around how to deal with vomiting incidents seemed an extreme version of the other daily procedures that Ladybird staff dealt with when feeding the children, and which allowed for less flexibility in how staff might bring their own ethics of care into the situation.

"They're always changing that rule": competing ethics of care within an institutional context

Tronto argues that, because care is multifaceted and especially complex when institutionalised as paid labour, there is always a possibility for conflict to arise in caring practices (1993, 109). This is particularly important when discussing food and feeding which are crucial channels through which emotions and social unity are expressed.

For example, in the ethnography about residential childcare in Scotland quoted earlier, Emond et al. discuss the contradictory meaning that food can acquire in institutional settings, being both an expression of care but also a channel through which power and resistance are enacted (2014, 1843). Aside from providing adequately for the children, staff members were also under pressure to not breach codes of practice or blur the boundaries of the relationship between themselves and the children, which needed to be 'familiar' but not intimate. Meals thus became a time and space of tension for both children and adults in this context, a domain of institutional life to be kept under control.

In the context of a Danish childcare setting, Hansen and Kristensen (2017) also discuss the tensions between the emotional dimension of food and some of the aims that childcare workers were trying to achieve when feeding children. Whilst staff members recognised the caring and pleasurable quality of feeding, they also needed to balance these aspects of feeding children with guidelines and norms about the adequate food types and portion sizes they should serve at school (ibid., 492). Yet, there was no consensus on which nutritional issue should predominantly be addressed in this setting; some staff prioritised helping children to develop "healthy tastes" (ibid., 495), others helped children with "small appetites" (ibid., 492) to eat more, or try different foods.

Similar situations arose at Ladybird when there was no consensus among staff about what was best practice during mealtimes, since colleagues seemed to have different priorities in terms of their aims when feeding children. As mentioned, lunchtime was the most logistically complex mealtime in the nursery, and required a lot of coordination, of the children as well as between staff. When I asked Joanne what she thought the most important aspect of her job was during a semi-structured interview, she replied:

> *Just making sure that everything...that the timing's right, that everyone's got a seat...also, the hygiene on site, in the kitchen, making sure everything is clean. Encouraging the children to eat, and sit right, and all them kind of things – semi-structured interview, July 2017.*

Although Joanne referred to some of the aims already described above ('getting children to eat' and promoting table manners), she initially emphasised the logistical aspect of lunchtime. This was indeed something that Joanne paid more attention to compared to the other staff. In her daily practices, she was particularly aware and concerned that lunchtime food deliveries were on time and that Mary, the cook who brought in the food trolleys into the nursery, also followed the lunchtime schedule properly. Joanne's frustration when things did not go to plan was particularly evident, for instance, over a time period when Mary was on sick leave and a temporary cook was hired who Joanne, and other staff members, did not think fulfilled the role to the same standards as Mary. These views seemed to be shared by others. In the following excerpts from my fieldnotes I noted:

> *Half-way through lunch, Charlene, the temp cook, comes in to speak to Joanne to ask about dessert. The food provider did not bring custard today so she's wondering whether she should make it herself using the custard powder available in the kitchen. Joanne says the cake will have to be served on its own because "it's too late to make the custard now." Joanne seems a bit annoyed; after Charlene leaves the room she complains to me that she still doesn't know where anything is, and is "constantly seeking reassurance" – fieldnotes, November 2016.*

> *Today for dessert we have berry compote and yoghurt. After Charlene distributes the food to each table, Grace [nursery teacher] and Stacey [lunchtime assistant] mention that Mary used to serve the compote inside the metal trays, and Grace asks herself out loud why they are now being served in jugs (as if to imply that the temp cook is not serving the food in the right way) – fieldnotes, December 2016.*

These indirect ways of communicating disagreements were prevalent, and were also voiced with regards to what and how children were fed. One day when I was assisting Fatima at the lunch table, she started passing the bread plate to the children while we waited for food to arrive, so that they could have a slice while we waited. Passing through our classroom, Joanne said to Fatima it was better to not give them bread so that they would not fill up on it before their meal. Fatima shared her frustration with me when Joanne was out of earshot: "*They're always changing that rule, one day we can, the other we can't, it's so confusing. I don't actually know what we're meant to do.*"

Whilst several staff members were largely invested in promoting healthy eating and table manners (like Robert and Ruby), or were particularly attentive to the logistical aspects of feeding children (like Joanne), others were also concerned with making mealtimes convivial and pleasurable occasions for children. Staff members' flexibility when taking children's viewpoints into account varied. For example, earlier I noted Joyce's views about the contrast between mealtimes and the rest of the day's activities, which were a lot more child-led. Similarly, tea-club was a space in which staff's various aims and approaches were most evident, as it was set up in different ways depending on which staff member was running it. When I started fieldwork in August 2016, a young woman called Sandra was in charge of tea-club. She emphasised conviviality in her sessions. She tried to follow the suggested menu as closely as possible, and never talked to children about nutritional facts. The only conversations she and the children had about food were about what they wanted to eat. Sandra would tell them what was on the menu, and if one of the children said they did not want that day's meal, she would try to modify the dish so that everyone would be happy with their supper.

After Sandra left this job, Joyce took over the sessions. She had a similar attitude to Sandra's, not seeing mealtimes as an opportunity to educate the children but rather to spend quality time together, even referring to tea-club as a "family" on several occasions. As Hansen and Kristensen have argued for their case study in Denmark, "To be shown consideration for one's [food] preferences is one way of practicing care" (2017, 491). People's different approaches when feeding children within Ladybird are important examples of how institutionalised caregiving can be understood as contradictory. These show that some of the mechanisms which are in place for carework to be carried out 'effectively' also determine whether the kind of care given is considered acceptable practice or not, depending on how close practitioners might stay to specific bureaucratic guidelines. As mentioned, these tensions could add some strain to the work relationships between staff. For instance, during our semi-structured interview, Robert expressed that achieving the 'outcomes' he considered desirable for what children were fed at tea-club were dependent on staff members' commitment to preparing food:

> *What we're able to charge parents doesn't meet anywhere near the cost of running [tea club], and there's no support from the local authority in running an extended day service. So thinking about what do you provide, and with really no budget, is tough. What I would like to do, there isn't the money for that [and] the practicalities and the reality of preparing something fairly complex from scratch, there isn't really the time [...] But interestingly I think depending on the member of staff running it [tea club] was about how successful the children were in eating or not eating. So, initially at some point there was quite a resistance from the members of staff in making a simple lentil soup that can be made in a matter of minutes. So because they were quite... I wouldn't say against it, but they didn't like it, their beliefs were projected onto the children and therefore the children didn't like it. I never really got full assessment on whether that was the member of staff's point of view or whether the children didn't really like it. Or was it...that it takes a bit of time and effort, whereas whacking something in the oven is very simple. So I think that came into it, because with different members of staff there were different levels of success we were able to achieve – semi-structured interview, August 2017.*

Robert's account sheds light on the competing views among staff about what the priorities of feeding children at Ladybird are, but also the tension between bureaucratic universalism and the particularism of caring practices. The words he chooses, such as not having had a "full assessment" about the "success" of given approaches, also mirror the way in which the language of policy and audit culture (Power 1999; Strathern 2000; Shore 2017) play out in the everyday lives of childcare workers. At the same time, the issues he identifies, such as lack of funding to provide the food he believes is adequate, and the varying level of skill that staff have, points to some of the contradictions already discussed about the ECEC policy landscape. On the one hand, the early years are framed as a crucial time in children's lives, in which important developmental and educational goals are to be achieved (Moss and Petrie 2000; Penn 2011). On the other, childcare continues to be an undervalued occupation in England, in which the workforce is often over-worked and underpaid; early years food policy (not being statutory) offers voluntary guidelines to settings, which can be adhered to or not depending on the various material restrictions in each context. In this sense, the constraints staff faced in providing care are very much structural rather than simply shaped by each person's experiences and knowledge.

Notes

1 Considered 'healthy options' by the staff at Ladybird, and marketed as such. Weetabix is a popular whole-grain wheat cereal produced in the U.K. Rice Krispies is a toasted rice cereal produced by the American brand Kellogg's – neither contain added sugars.
2 This usually consists of breadsticks, toast, rice cakes, or plain tortilla chips (corn-based crisp).
3 Similarly, Mechling sees children's food play (both with 'imagined' and real foods) as a way in which children "deconstruct culture" (2000, 21) and "as productive experimentation with what is pleasing to our eyes, noses, touch, and taste" (ibid., 22).
4 This is explored at length in Chapter 5.
5 This policy, introduced in September 2017, is discussed in the Introduction.
6 Provided to parents who were taking English for Speakers of Other Languages (ESOL) classes at Ladybird, in the training room adjacent to the children's centre.

References

Abel, Emily K., and Margaret K. Nelson. 1990. 'Circles of Care: An Introductory Essay'. In *Circles of Care: Work and Identity in Women's Life*, edited by Emily K. Abel and Margaret K. Nelson, 4–34. New York: State University of New York Press.

Afflerback, Sara, Shannon K. Carter, Amanda Koontz Anthony, and Liz Grauerholz. 2013. 'Infant-Feeding Consumerism in the Age of Intensive Mothering and Risk Society'. *Journal of Consumer Culture* 13 (3): 387–405. https://doi.org/10.1177/1469540513485271.

Albon, Deborah, and Anette Hellman. 2018. 'Of Routine Consideration: "Civilising" Children's Bodies via Food Events in Swedish and English Early Childhood Settings'. *Ethnography and Education*, January, 1–17. https://doi.org/10.1080/17457823.2017.1422985.

Baez, Benjamin, and Susan Talburt. 2008. 'Governing for Responsibility and with Love: Parents and Children between Home and School'. *Educational Theory* 58 (1): 25–43.

Bakhtin, Mikhail. 1986. *Speech Genres and other Late Essays*. Austin: University of Texas Press.

Beck, Ulrich. 1992. *Risk Society: Towards a New Modernity*. London: SAGE Publications.

Benn, Jette, and Monica Carlsson. 2014. 'Learning through School Meals?' *Appetite* 78 (July): 23–31. https://doi.org/10.1016/j.appet.2014.03.008.

Brooker, Liz. 2010. 'Constructing the Triangle of Care: Power and Professionalism in Practitioner/Parent Relationships'. *British Journal of Educational Studies* 58 (2): 181–96. https://doi.org/10.1080/00071001003752203.

Camps, Laura, and Tony Long. 2012. 'Origins, Purpose and Future of Sure Start Children's Centres'. *Nursing Children and Young People* 24 (1): 26–30.

Children's Food Trust. 2012. 'Eat Better Start Better Voluntary Food and Drink Guidelines for Early Years Settings in England – A Practical Guide'. Sheffield: Children's Food Trust.

http://media.childrensfoodtrust.org.uk/2015/06/CFT_Early_Years_Guide_Interactive_ Sept-12.pdf.

Clarke, Karen. 2006. 'Childhood, Parenting and Early Intervention: A Critical Examination of the Sure Start National Programme'. *Critical Social Policy* 26 (4): 699–721. https:// doi.org/10.1177/0261018306068470.

Crozier, Gill. 1998. 'Parents and Schools: Partnership or Surveillance?' *Journal of Education Policy* 13 (1): 125–36. https://doi.org/10.1080/0268093980130108.

Dahlberg, Gunilla, and Peter Moss. 2004. *Ethics and Politics in Early Childhood Education*. London: Routledge.

Department for Education. 2017. 'Statutory Framework for the Early Years Foundation Stage: Setting the Standards for Learning, Development and Care for Children from Birth to Five'. London: Department for Education. https://assets.publishing.service. gov.uk/government/uploads/system/uploads/attachment_data/file/596629/EYFS_ STATUTORY_FRAMEWORK_2017.pdf.

Donzelot, Jaques. 1977. *The Policing of Families*. London: The John Hopkins University Press.

Elias, Norbert. 1994. *The Civilizing Process*. Oxford: Blackwell Publishing Ltd.

Elliott, Charlene. 2010. 'Eatertainment and the (Re)Classification of Children's Foods'. *Food, Culture & Society* 13 (4): 539–53. https://doi.org/10.2752/175174410X12777254289385.

Emond, Ruth, Ian McIntosh, and Samantha Punch. 2014. 'Food and Feelings in Residential Childcare'. *British Journal of Social Work* 44 (7): 1840–56. https://doi.org/10.1093/bjsw/ bct009.

England, Paula. 2005. 'Emerging Theories of Care Work'. *Annual Review of Sociology* 31 (1): 381–99. https://doi.org/10.1146/annurev.soc.31.041304.122317.

England, Paula, and Nancy Folbre. 1999. 'The Cost of Caring'. *Annals of the American Academy of Political and Social Science* 561 (January): 39–51.

Faircloth, Charlotte. 2014. 'Intensive Parenting and the Expansion of Parenting'. In *Parenting Culture Studies*, edited by Ellie Lee, Jennie Bristow, Charlotte Faircloth, and Jan Macvarish, 25–50. Basingstoke: Palgrave Macmillan.

Fischler, Claude. 2011. 'Commensality, society and culture.' *Social Science Information* 50 (3–4): 528–48. https://doi.org/10.1177/0539018411413963

Flowers, Rick, and Elaine Swan, eds. 2016. *Food Pedagogies*. London: Routledge.

Foucault, Michel. 1991. 'Governmentality'. In *The Foucault Effect: Studies in Governmentality, with Two Lectures by and an Interview with Michel Foucault*, edited by Graham Burchell, Colin Gordon, and Peter Miller, 87–104. Chicago: University of Chicago Press.

Gullberg, Eva. 2006. 'Food for Future Citizens: School Meal Culture in Sweden'. *Food, Culture and Society: An International Journal of Multidisciplinary Research* 9 (3): 337– 43. https://doi.org/10.2752/155280106778813279.

Hansen, Stine Rosenlund, and Niels Heine Kristensen. 2017. 'Food for Kindergarten Children: Who Cares? Relations between Food and Care in Everyday Kindergarten Mealtime'. *Food, Culture & Society* 20 (3): 485–502. https://doi.org/10.1080/1552801 4.2017.1288783.

Leahy, Deana, and Peta Malins. 2015. 'Biopedagogical Assemblages: Exploring School Drug Education in Action'. *Cultural Studies? Critical Methodologies* 15 (5): 398–406.

Lupton, Deborah. 1996. *Food, the Body and the Self*. London: SAGE Publications.

Maher, JaneMaree, Suzanne Fraser, and Jan Wright. 2010. 'Framing the Mother: Childhood Obesity, Maternal Responsibility and Care'. *Journal of Gender Studies* 19 (3): 233–47. https://doi.org/10.1080/09589231003696037.

Michel, S. 2002. 'Afterword: Dilemmas of Childcare'. In *Child Care Policy at the Crossroads. Gender and Welfare State Restructuring*, edited by R. Mahon and S. Michel, 333–338. New York: Routlegde.

Mol, Annemarie. 2008. *The Logic of Care: Health and the Problem of Patient Choice*. London: Routledge.

Moran-Ellis, Jo. 2010. 'Reflections on the Sociology of Childhood in the UK'. *Current Sociology* 58 (2): 186–205. https://doi.org/10.1177/0011392109354241.

Moss, Peter. 2012. 'Poor, Consumer, Citizen? What Image of the Parent in England?' *Rivista Italiana Di Educazione Familiare* 1: 63–78.

Moss, Peter, and Pat Petrie. 2000. *From Children's Services to Children's Spaces*. London: Routledge/Falmer.

Murphy, Elizabeth. 2000. 'Risk, Responsibility and Rhetoric in Infant Feeding'. *Journal of Contemporary Ethnography* 29 (3): 291–325.

Ofsted. 2015. 'Early Years and Childcare Registration Handbook'. Manchester: Ofsted. https://www.gov.uk/government/publications/become-a-registered-early-years-or-childcare-provider-in-england.

Penn, Helen. 2011. 'Policy Rationales for Early Childhood Services'. *International Journal of Child Care and Education Policy* 5 (1): 1–16. https://doi.org/10.1007/2288-6729-5-1-1.

Petherick, LeAnne. 2015. 'Shaping the Child as a Healthy Child: Health Surveillance, Schools, and Biopedagogies'. *Cultural Studies? Critical Methodologies* 15 (5): 361–70.

Pike, Jo, and Deana Leahy. 2012. 'School Food and the Pedagogies of Parenting'. *Australian Journal of Adult Learning* 52 (3): 434.

Powell, Martin. 2014. *Understanding the Mixed Economy of Welfare*. Bristol: The Policy Press.

Power, Michael. 1999. *The Audit Society: Rituals of Verification*. Oxford: Oxford University Press.

Rafalovich, Adam. 2013. 'Attention Deficit-Hyperactivity Disorder as the Medicalization of Childhood: Challenges from and for Sociology'. *Sociology Compass* 7 (5): 343–54. https://doi.org/10.1111/soc4.12034.

Sayer, Andrew. 2017. 'Responding to the Troubled Families Programme: Framing the Injuries of Inequality'. *Social Policy and Society* 16 (01): 155–64. https://doi.org/10.1017/S1474746416000373.

Shore, Cris. 2017. 'Audit Culture and the Politics of Responsibility: Beyond Neoliberal Responsibilization?' In *Competing Responsibilities: The Ethics and Politics of Contemporary Life*, edited by Susanna Trnka and Catherine Trundle, 96–117. Durham: Duke University Press.

Strathern, Marylin. 2000. 'Introduction: New Accountabilities'. In *Audit Cultures: Anthropological Studies in Accountability, Ethics and the Academy*, edited by Marylin Strathern, 1–18. London: Routledge.

Tronto, Joan C. 1993. *Moral Boundaries: A Political Argument for an Ethic of Care*. New York: Routlegde.

———. 2013. 'Introduction: When Care Is No Longer "at Home"'. In *Caring Democracy. Markets, Equality, and Justice*, 1–16. New York: New York University Press.

Van Krieken, Robert. 1998. *Norbert Elias*. London: Routledge.

White, E. Jayne. 2017. 'A Feast of Fools: Mealtimes as Democratic Acts of Resistance and Collusion in Early Childhood Education'. *Knowledge Cultures* 5 (3): 85. https://doi.org/10.22381/KC5320177.

Wiley, Andrea S., and John S. Allen. 2013. *Medical Anthropology: A Biocultural Approach*. New York: Oxford University Press.

4 Children's eating practices in childcare

The previous chapter examined the bureaucratic and practical demands of feeding children at Ladybird through the accounts of staff members and my own participant observation. Having contextualised how mealtimes were organised on a day-to-day basis, as well as exploring the various (and at times competing) aims that staff pursued when feeding children, this chapter now turns to an analysis of children's experiences from the children's point of view.

Following Corsaro's work on 'interpretive reproduction,' this chapter asks: how do children create self- and peer-group identities through food and eating practices within a childcare setting? I argue that group unity was achieved through play behaviour, humour, and role reversal. Following the work of Nolas, Varvantakis, and Aruldoss (2017, 2018) on 'idioms of childhood,' I also ask: what do children consider meaningful about food and mealtimes? Drawing from these authors, I contend that children's role-play, drawings, and other forms of expression are valid representations of what children deemed meaningful about food and eating practices. Through these various 'idioms,' children represented (and performed) food and mealtimes as channels through which to express care, enact authority, and communicate their knowledge (both child- and adult-centred) about food and social relationships.

Finally, as well as focusing on children's voices, this chapter will also delve into their exchanges with adults during mealtimes, and some of the viewpoints about these daily routines that the school staff shared with me. Thus, the chapter also explores the question: how do children negotiate power relations with school staff during mealtimes? I will explore how the work of social philosopher and cultural theorist Mikhail Bakhtin on the 'dialogic' (1986) and the carnivalesque (1968) may complement Corsaro's notions about interpretive reproduction (2011), adding to our understanding of how children's knowledge and sense of self is produced co-relationally, through their engagement with the multiple social worlds that they inhabit.

Meaningful mealtimes: peer cultures, humour, and play behaviour

In the previous chapter, I described the daily mealtime routines at Ladybird to provide a detailed insight of the logistical aspects of mealtimes, and how this shaped staff members' practices. I now turn to an exploration of how children

DOI: 10.4324/9781003297642-5

created unity during meals, and what they seemed to consider meaningful about food and eating within these institutional constraints.

The regulation of daily activities, including mealtimes, is part and parcel of how control and surveillance are enacted (to various degrees) within institutions (e.g. Goffman 1968). Whilst at Ladybird there could certainly be a lot of flexibility in how some of the mealtimes were coordinated, as will be shown, these moments also stood out as the times during which children were most encouraged to actively learn in a concentrated manner – differently to the rest of the day's activities, which were more child-led. Drawing from Corsaro's work on interpretive reproduction (2011) and that of Nolas, Varvantakis, and Aruldoss on 'idioms of childhood' (2017, 2018), I will particularly explore how humour and play behaviour played an important role in peer cultures, both to promote conviviality, create meaning, and contest adult norms and rules. Of particular influence to this analysis is Bakhtin's work on the 'dialogic' (1986), which has been increasingly applied in studies about Early Childhood Education and Care (ECEC) contexts (Albon and Rosen 2014; Marjanovic-Shane and White 2014; White 2014; Tallant 2015; Tallant 2017; Cohen 2017), also to specifically examine mealtime interactions in these settings (White 2017).

> *After hanging her coat and washing her hands, Crystal [four years-old] sits next to me at the table and asks Ruby for toast with honey: she tells me it's her "favourite." I ask her if she also eats toast with honey at home and she says no. I ask, "What do you have for breakfast at home then?" and she says, "Shreddies,[1] with no milk," and giggles whilst checking, with a side-glance, if Ruby heard her (I assume she does this because she thinks Ruby might tell her it's unusual to eat cereal without any milk). I tell her that when I was a little girl I also didn't like to eat my cereal with milk in it, and I also didn't like drinking cold milk. I ask her, "Do you think that's weird?" She giggles again and says, "Yes!" – fieldnotes, February 2017.*

On most days, breakfast club was a quiet time at Ladybird. Children who attended breakfast club and tea-club were trusted to "be more independent," in the words of the staff, so were allowed and encouraged to help themselves to milk or water from the jugs on their table, as well as the food provided.

In these morning and afternoon sessions, children openly monitored each other's behaviour and preferences, often assuming an adult-like role when doing so, and expressing what they thought was right or wrong about each other's food practices, showing an awareness of staff members' expectations. For instance, they reminded each other to say "please" and "thank you" when asking for food, a task that was pervasive among the staff, alongside the frequent reminders to "be kind to each other" and the repetition of "sharing is caring."[2] Children tested the boundaries of what was deemed acceptable by the adults in a number of ways: in subtle remarks, such as Crystal's secretive admission to me that she liked to eat cereal without milk, as described above, or in more open and transgressive ways, such as eating with one's hands instead of using cutlery. Children also claimed some authority during mealtimes through role reversal. In my adoption of a 'least adult role' (Mandell 1988;

Warming 2005) in my research, I also complied when children asked me to lend them my visitor's badge. When this happened, they would 'become' me, and I the child who had my badge, which then meant they would boss me around a little, either telling me to wash my hands or also eat what was being served to them. My aim of embodying a 'least adult' role is also a response to my desire to engage in children's play "as an ideologue" (Marjanovic-Shane and White 2014, 123) rather than as an unengaged participant – by being responsive to the meanings that children created and conveyed through playful behaviour and humour.

The adoption of an adult or authoritative role by children can be understood as an act of what Corsaro has described as 'interpretive reproduction' (2011). The term, which Corsaro coined to theorise children's collective participation in society, is defined as follows:

> The term *interpretive* captures the innovative and creative aspects of children's participation in society…children create and participate in their own unique peer cultures by creatively taking or appropriating information from the adult world to address their own peer concerns. The term *reproduction* captures the idea that children are not simply internalizing society and culture but are actively contributing to cultural production and change.
>
> (ibid., 20–21, original emphasis)

At Ladybird I observed that through role reversal, children *reproduced* some of the behaviours they perceived from the adult world by embodying an authoritative position. Simultaneously, their *interpretation* of these attitudes was a way in which children responded and reacted to their 'peer concerns' by taking some of the control and management of mealtimes into their own hands, making them a playful and convivial occasion.

Such acts of resistance performed by children were a way to subvert adults' control, yet also a way to establish unity, and express group belonging and empathy. Showing that they knew what others liked was another way in which this manifested itself, as children could position their knowledge above that of the adults. One morning, for example, when Ruby asked Eva (four-years-old) what she'd like for breakfast, Crystal answered instead of her, saying enthusiastically, "She's a Rice Krispies girl!" – as indeed Eva was, since this was always her choice of breakfast food during the time I spent at Ladybird. Similar moments were also common during the more logistically complex and formal lunch hours. Once, while one of the lunchtime assistants was serving food for the group she and I were sitting with, Amir (four-years-old) very decisively told her what she should give his friend Timur (also four): "He likes chicken, and baked potato, and salad!" These instances, as well being examples of how children established unity with each other, showed children's awareness of each other's individualised identities around food preferences, which not all staff might have recognised to the same degree, or validated equally if trying to encourage children to try different foods.

Peer groups were often perceived as a potentially positive 'influence' on individual children's eating by both staff and parents. For instance, the propensity for children to eat new kinds of foods (or foods they claimed to dislike) when they ate with friends was deemed particularly valuable. Parents would often express surprise that their child had eaten a particular food that, they said, 'they would never eat at home.' In fact, children were often curious about what the people around them were having, and conversations about what different foods tasted like often resulted in children trying something new. However, whilst children at times encouraged each other to try different things because they liked the taste, commensality also played a big role in children's daily experience of mealtimes at Ladybird. Fischler describes commensality as not exclusively restricted to special or ritual occasions, but more so as an essential component of our daily meals (2011, 531). Thus, as well as adding to the exploration of eating – beyond its nutritional function – as a fundamental way in which collective identities are formed (Fischler 1988, 280), children's commensality at the nursery also invited me to assess the limitations of adults' involvement in shaping children's daily practices.

Elliott's reflections about 'eatertainment' (2010) – the emergence of commercialised 'fun' foods for children – also prove useful here. She argues that children are not deceived by the tactics of 'eatertainment' but rather active agents in this process of making food and eating 'fun,' making food play meaningful for themselves and their peers (2010, 546). Whilst it is adults that often control *what* children eat, whether it is via advertising, within families, or institutional settings, it is also important to note that children determine *how* they eat. In this way, children create their own norms and behaviours about food and eating, establishing a common meaning among them, and also subverting adult control (to some degree), as has also been noted by Marjanovic-Shane and White (2014). Group identity was emphasised in new mealtime norms promoted among children, in a manner similar to that in which adults communicated the standards they wanted children to abide by. For instance, rules were created about how certain foods should be eaten. A recurrent case was that of the berry compote and Greek yogurt dessert option at lunch, which children infallibly instructed each other to mix, "*to make it pink.*" On an occasion during which I chose this option for dessert, Crystal was puzzled when she saw I kept the compote and yogurt separate rather than mixing them, and asked me if she could mix my pudding for me, to which I agreed. During tea-club, if spaghetti was being served, children would very often dangle the pasta above their faces from their forks and into their mouths, a technique which was predictably not greatly appreciated by the staff members, yet one through which the children bonded by exhibiting each other's ability to eat spaghetti in this way.

Indeed, many of the instances I observed highlighted that whilst adults tended to focus on *what* children ate, it was *how* they spent a mealtime together (whether they could partake in the activity as a group) that seemed to matter more to children, and adults often had less control over this. An example was an occasion in which I was helping the lunchtime assistants by sitting with Simon, a four-year-old boy with special needs.[3] In the months that I spent getting to know him, Simon never seemed to like having lunch at Ladybird, and days on which the staff succeeded in persuading him to sit with the other children were a cause for celebration. This alone was perceived as a victory, since Simon was unwilling and, to a considerable extent, also physically unable to eat the food provided at the nursery; his mother told us that, due to complications after being born prematurely, he had difficulties consuming solid meals, so his diet at home still consisted primarily of pureed foods.[4] The main difficulty for him was the texture and consistency of solid foods; on an occasion in which Simon tried to eat some rice during lunchtime, for example, he was unable to swallow, so started choking and ultimately threw up on his plate.

One of the aims of him attending lunch at Ladybird once a week, on Tuesdays, was to introduce him to different kinds of foods and it was hoped that eating with children his age would provide encouragement. On this particular day when I was asked to sit with him, Simon was more distressed than usual when the time to have lunch came. As he often did, he cried intensely and refused to sit on his chair, so I held him on my lap to comfort him. At one point during this episode, he refused to continue sitting on my legs and laid down on the floor; as this was unfolding and the lunchtime assistant and I looked to each other concernedly, Johnny (three-years-old), who was sitting to the left of Simon and I, leaned towards him and affectionately patted Simon on the head. After this brief interaction, Simon stopped crying and sat on his own chair, next to Johnny, and lunch continued without further disruption.

Unity and comradeship were thus evident during meals, but also during the games children played in the 'kitchen corner,' in which friendships were reinforced, and where exclusion was also a potential threat – indeed, as with 'real' food practices. As well as observing these games, I was also often invited to partake in them:

> *After snack time, Crystal goes to the kitchen corner and asks me to come over; she pulls a chair out from under the little table and tells me, "Fran I'm going to cook you something." She starts filling one of the toy metal bowls with different food-shaped toys. "First these ingredients," she says, as she puts an orange, a piece of cheese, and some cherries inside the bowl. She then places the metal bowl under the toy electric whisk, and she brings it over to me so I can assist her. After we are done 'mixing' the ingredients, she takes the bowl to the microwave saying, "This is a warm oven," as she puts the bowl inside it. While the food 'cooks,' she brings me the toy milk carton with a cup and says, "Here's a bit of milk." Moments later, she extracts the bowl from the oven and brings it to me, adding, "Let me give you something [cutlery] to eat with." I ask her, "What is this?" and she says, "Bolognese sauce!" I 'eat' saying how delicious it is. In the meantime, she grabs two toy telephones, and gives one to me. She puts her receiver next to her ear and makes a ringing sound, which is the signal that tells me I should answer my phone. I pick up, and after we say hello to each other, I ask Crystal where she is: "At home," she says. "What are you doing?" I ask: "Making dinner for a friend!" she replies. She ends the conversation by 'hanging up.' She then asks me, "Did you enjoy it [your dinner]?" and I tell her I enjoyed it very much, thanking her – fieldnotes, April 2017.*

It was common for me to take part in interactions like these that, I maintain, provided me with valuable insights into children's viewpoints about the function of eating practices, and through which children were able to communicate their preferences on their own terms. Following the work of Nolas, Varvantakis, and Aruldoss (2017, 2018), in my research I consider play as an "idiom of childhood," a concept that defines the different modes of communication that children make use of as meaningful representations of their knowledge and perspectives. Through the multi-methods, child-centred approach I adopted in my fieldwork, this exchange in the kitchen corner with Crystal became part of a broader conversation she and I had been having, in the months we spent together, about her eating habits at home and school. During a drawing activity, when I asked if she could draw one of her favourite foods on a paper plate, she drew – what she explained was – spaghetti Bolognese (Figure 4.1), which she said she liked to eat with her mother. This, paired with our 'phone conversation' above, in which Crystal expressed that she was "*making dinner for a friend*," suggested to me that she might find this dish a particularly comforting food, and one that she would want to share with people she cares for.

Role-play (which I also consider an idiom of childhood) was another medium through which children reproduced and communicated family roles, as they knew them from their own daily lives. One morning, I was invited to have 'breakfast' in the 'kitchen corner' by Lucy (four-years-old), who gave me some 'fruit' and 'yoghurt,' whilst Crystal and Eva poured me 'coffee.' Searching through the toy

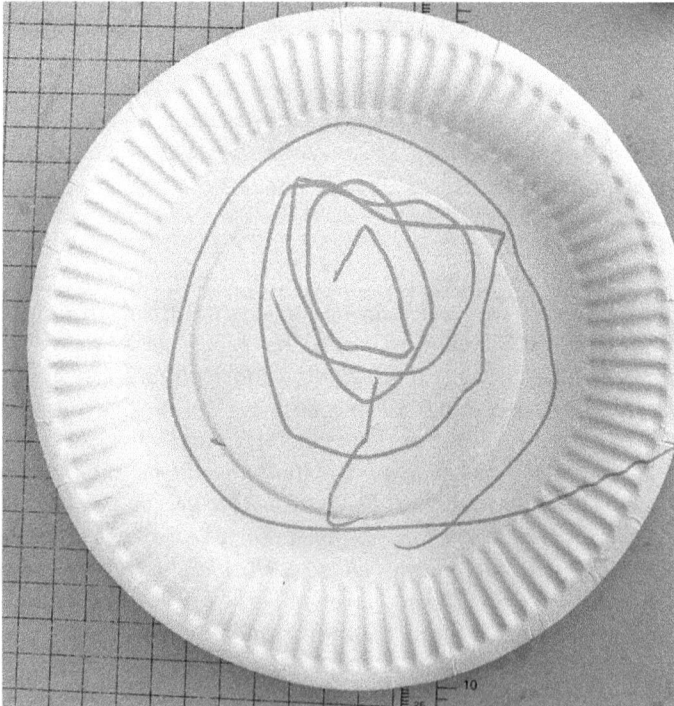

Figure 4.1 'Spaghetti Bolognese' – Crystal (4).
Photograph by the author.

box, Lucy asked, "Where is the croissant?" and after finding it and handing it to me she said that we should rush – "I have to get to work!" she exclaimed – and instructed me to wrap my toy croissant in a napkin so I could "save it for later." This request seemed to mirror Lucy's and her mother's morning routine, of which the staff and I had glimpses when Lucy was dropped off to breakfast club in the mornings. Lucy's mother, a single parent working full time, would often comment on her daily time constraints, and the difficulty of getting Lucy ready quickly in the mornings. This would at times result in her bringing what Lucy was having for breakfast at home to the children's centre, for her to finish eating after being dropped off.

Through play behaviour, I also learnt that 'preparing' and 'cooking' food was particularly important to children – both boys and girls – when playing in the kitchen corner, and that 'cooking' was often performed as a social and collaborative act. All the toy utensils provided to them were enthusiastically used to mimic the different actions of cutting, mixing, stirring, etc. A common theme was that of 'cutting' fruits and vegetables before 'serving' them, as illustrated in the fieldnotes below:

> *After Eva is done eating [breakfast] she goes to the kitchen corner and plays with a 'baby' [doll]; Crystal and I are still at the table. Eva lays out some 'breakfast foods' on the doll's chair, which Crystal questions jokingly: "A sausage for breakfast? And a watermelon? All these ingredients will make the baby fat!" Eva giggles and goes back to the toy basket and gets an 'apple.' Crystal tells her, "An apple?! You have to cut it first!" Eva pulls out a wooden knife from the drawer to 'chop' the fruit – fieldnotes, March 2017.*

Preparing food, or cooking, was an activity that children seemed to associate with adult behaviour and care, and which gave them authority during role-play. Whereas eating was predominantly perceived as children's practice, cooking and feeding others was seen as a role for grown-ups. As Tessa (four-years-old) once said to Sima, one of the lunchtime assistants, when she asked her if she "made cake at home": *"No, because I'm not a grown-up yet!"*

The negotiations that happened between children during mealtimes and food games provided them with opportunities to perform the act of sharing food as a caring and unifying practice. Simultaneously, these were moments during which children could express their knowledge about food and eating, and in which they recreated and communicated the norms that they were being encouraged to follow by adults. Viewing role-play as an idiom of childhood (Nolas, Varvantakis, and Aruldoss 2018) thus provided an insight into how interpretive reproduction (Corsaro 2011) happens in practice. Crystal's concern with Eva's choices of breakfast foods for the doll, although expressed humorously, showed an attempt to communicate some of the notions about healthy eating that the school staff promoted. Similar to children's covert and overt acts of resistance during mealtimes, role-playing and food games provided them with a platform to test the boundaries of the norms they knew, and negotiate positions of authority based on this knowledge.

Disrupted food cultures

Of course, it was also not always the case that children were able to equally partake in all the food practices (both 'real' and playful) that took place at Ladybird. An extreme example is that of Cindy (four-years-old). The school staff were asked by her mother to not include her in any mainstream holiday celebrations, such as Christmas, Halloween, or Easter, because of their religious denomination. On occasions when children were taking part in events related to such festivities, Cindy would sit in the children's centre where other members of staff or I would read her a book, or play with her. One time during which Cindy had to step away from her class, who were listening to Christmas carols, Cindy reflected on why she could not partake in this activity, explaining to me that she knew she could not celebrate Christmas "*because*," she said, "*it would make [religious figure] sad.*"

A more difficult episode took place in March, before the Easter term break. During tea-club, I brought in a basket of chocolate eggs from the staff room that one of the teachers had put aside for the 'tea-clubbers.' I was distributing these to the children, and after I gave one to Cindy, Ruby told me that Cindy was not meant to eat any Easter eggs because of her religion, and I was asked to take it back from her. Asking Cindy to put the egg back in the basket was perhaps one of the most difficult moments I faced during fieldwork, both because I knew that this would be very upsetting for Cindy, and because I did not feel like I could challenge Ruby's instructions that I do this. Although I tried to explain to Cindy that I was taking the egg back because her mother had asked us to, this moment deeply upset her, and the 'least adult role' (Mandell 1988; Warming 2005) that I had been trying to maintain as much as possible no longer felt legitimate. Ultimately, however, this event did not cause any damage to Cindy's and my relationship. She never mentioned the incident to me again, and our interactions continued as they had before.

Other moments of exclusion were related to dietary restrictions, also due to religion or allergies. One boy, Andrew (three-years-old) who was intolerant to gluten was not able to eat pizza for supper one afternoon, which also upset him, and Ruby's and Joyce's explanations that the school did not have the 'special' pizza that he ate at home – as his mother had told us – did not comfort him. Other children's reactions when others became sad or otherwise distressed were often to reach out to one another, as already exemplified above in the lunchtime interaction between Simon and Johnny. Questions would also ensue, both to the children whose eating was different and, if they were unable or unwilling to answer, to the staff members.

Negotiating power relations: food as a pedagogical tool

Food has already been identified as a complex and multifaceted entity in children's daily life at Ladybird. Beyond providing nutrition, its role in children's sociality with each other and adults, as well as its use in play behaviour to appropriate and recreate adults' roles and norms, has also been discussed as a way in which interpretive reproduction (Corsaro 2011) happens in practice. However, exploring how children engage with food when childcare practitioners employ it as a pedagogical tool (Flowers and Swan 2016) is also important. As I argued in Chapter 3, at Ladybird food and meals were used as pedagogical tools in several ways: to teach children about 'healthy eating,' to teach them about table manners, and to overcome 'fussy eating.' Further, nutritional knowledge was at times tied together to notions about bodily appearance, which links to Lupton's premise that eating habits and manners are intertwined with notions of what constitutes a 'civilised self' (1996, 22). This was evident, for example, in an interaction between Ruby and Lucy one morning:

> *Crystal has drunk several glasses of milk during breakfast, as she usually does, which Ruby comments on, asking her whether she's not had too much already. Crystal says that she wants lots of milk so she can "be strong." Ruby asks Crystal if she knows why milk makes you strong; Crystal just says, "Because it makes you strong!" Ruby then explains that milk makes your bones strong, because it has calcium in it which helps the bones grow. She tells Crystal that she can feel the bones in her hands and her skull, showing her how to do this by pinching her own fingers and tapping her head.*
>
> *[A few days later, also at breakfast]*
>
> *After she is brought the toast she asked for, Crystal tells Ruby she wants honey to spread on the bread. Ruby tells her that she can't have honey every day because it has too much sugar, and "we shouldn't be eating a lot of sugar every day." Crystal asks, "Does sugar makes you strong like milk?" Ruby says it doesn't make you strong, and that it's bad for our teeth. Lucy arrives a bit later to breakfast club today; she also asks Ruby for toast and honey. Ruby tells her, "If you want honey you will have to have it tomorrow because..." and, looking at Crystal, she asks: "Why can't we have honey every day Crystal?" "Because it has too much sugar," she responds, "And why is that bad?" Ruby asks. Crystal doesn't reply. "Because it's bad for our teeth right?" says Ruby, also adding that, "Too much sugar is bad for our bodies." She then asks the entire group (Eva, Crystal, and Lucy) what we should do with our teeth every day, and Lucy says, "We need to wash them," "Yes," says Ruby, "We should brush our teeth every day." Lucy, next to whom I'm sitting, turns to me and says, "If you don't brush your teeth they become brown, and brown teeth are disgusting!" – fieldnotes, November 2016.*

Ruby's discussion about sugar avoidance touched on the impact that sugar can have on dental health; indeed, Lucy then expressed the unacceptability of having "brown teeth." When the topic of sugar was being discussed at the table, Ruby often used a model of the stages of tooth decay to explain to the children what she meant (Figure 4.2).

In exploring the embeddedness of nutrition and public health messages in children's daily practices at Ladybird, an interesting contradiction emerged. As alluded to earlier, whereas the rest of the activities, both at the nursery and the children's centre, followed a predominantly child-led, 'playing and learning,' model, mealtimes stood out as the only occasions when children were being actively taught

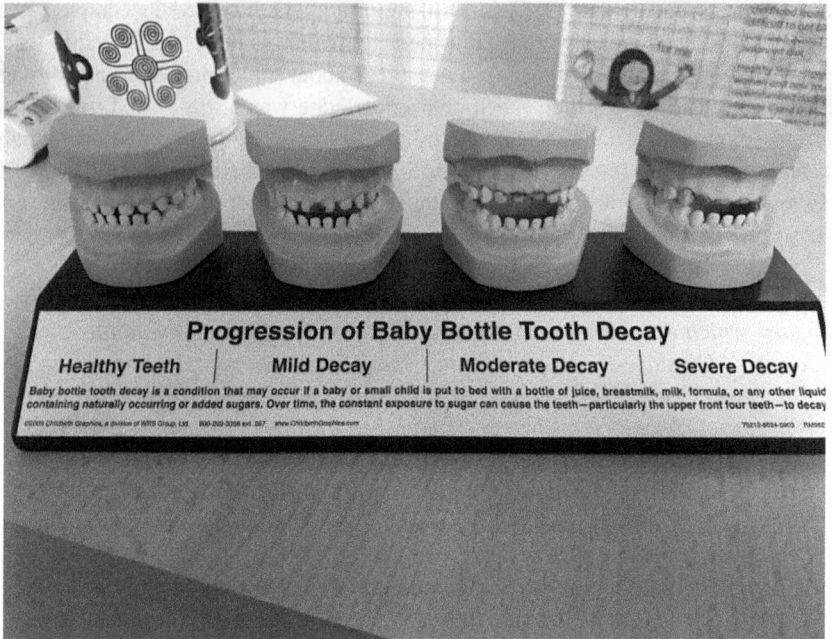

Figure 4.2 "Brown teeth are disgusting!"
Photograph by the author.

in a more systematic way, and during which their knowledge was tested on occasion, as also shown in other similar studies carried out in early years settings (e.g. Marjanovic-Shane and White 2014; Tallant 2015; White 2017). Joyce, in a semi-structured interview, discussed this paradox with me:

> They're here all day, they are doing an activity on the table and being encouraged to play with this, feel this, then they clear the table and put food on it, and they're told, "Don't play." But ten minutes ago they were playing on that table...so that to me, that's part of it, they have to play with their food [...] playing with their food, that's the first step that nobody wants to take, it's playing with their food...they tell parents even if they just lick it that's fine, but no, even if they play with it it's fine, that's the first step. So even at the snack table [in the children's centre] they're banging [plates] and parents say, "Don't bang, stop banging!" but...all we are doing is telling them to play except for this half an hour when they sit down with their food, that's insane. How are these kids supposed to know they're not playing now? – semi-structured interview, July 2017.

As discussed in Chapter 3, it was of course not the case that everyone shared Joyce's views about how children should conduct themselves during mealtimes. Nonetheless, her comment confirmed that there was indeed a discrepancy between this and other aspects of children's daily routine at Ladybird, and the potential for adults to empathise with children's viewpoints rather than always embodying a disciplining role. Joyce's account also shows that children's play might be understood differently by adults and children. Whilst for some staff children playing with their food might have been perceived as counter-productive, Joyce seemed to recognise that playing is a way by which children make sense of the phenomena around them and, as such, which should be taken seriously (White 2014; Nolas, Aruldoss, and Varvantakis 2018).

Nonetheless, as well as using play to make sense of mealtimes, there were a few ways in which children at Ladybird used play behaviour to respond – and resist – to food being used as a pedagogical tool during mealtimes. Play behaviour disrupted adults' attempts to engage in conversations about healthy eating, such as Ruby's advice on not eating too much sugar. In these moments, children could choose to turn the discussion into a playful debate. For example, when asked what vitamins certain fruits and vegetables had, or why the vitamin D and calcium contained in milk were good for them, children might deliberatively give a wrong (or 'silly') answer to challenge the adult talking to them.

Food and the dialogic (i): Bakhtin in children's peer groups

Corsaro has argued that investigating children's 'collective actions' is an important way to understand how agency and resistance are enacted, but also how children produce and participate in group cultures (2005). He describes collective actions as ways of behaving that are co-produced by children in relation to others (ibid., 213), through often repetitive actions. Several examples of these practices were evident at Ladybird: games involving food, like the spaghetti-dangling contest I described earlier or giving the wrong ('silly') answer to a question about food, can all be understood as collective actions. Children also made images on their plates with food (such as smiling faces or animal bodies, like in Figure 4.3), initiated 'food competitions' with each other,[5] or used breadsticks as 'vampire teeth'[6] – a game that I accidentally introduced early on during my fieldwork, and which caught on.[7]

This last practice in particular, which I inadvertently spread, made me reflect at length about the applicability of Mikhail Bakhtin's (1895–1975) work to childhood studies. Bakhtin, a social philosopher and cultural theorist working in 20th century Russia, is often most noted for his contributions in the field of literary criticism, although his intellectual legacy has been central to many other fields, including the social sciences (Gardiner and Mayerfeld Bell 1998, 14).

An important contribution by Bakhtin is his work on dialogism and the dialogic (1986), which serves as a basis from which to explore the relational and circular (or back-and-forth) nature of language – and human interaction. In Bakhtin's words, "Every one of our speech acts is influenced by previous experiences of language, and is constructed in consideration of the reactions we expect to obtain from our listener" (1986, 94). This circular vision of language is deemed particularly important by childhood studies scholars, such as White (2014), Albon and Rosen (2014), and Tobin et al. (2009), who pay special attention to the ways in which children's self and

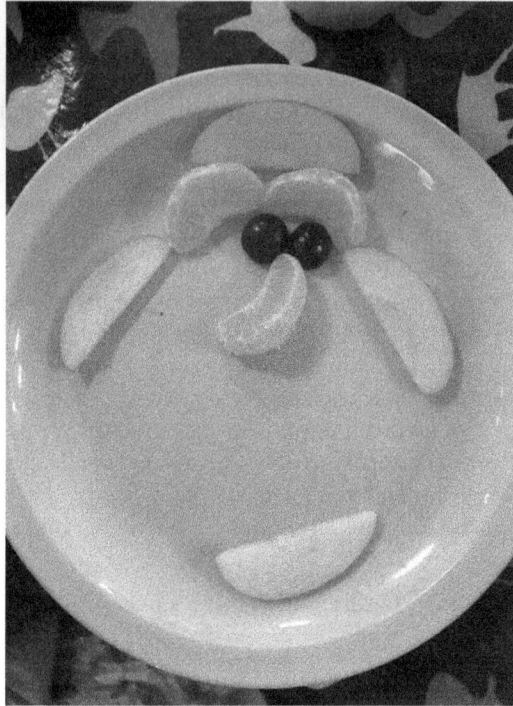

Figure 4.3 "An elephant on my plate!" – Crystal (4).

Photograph by the author.

group identities are created experientially and intersubjectively (i.e. in relation to and in response to others). Circular exchanges of words, gestures, and practices that the children playfully engaged in at Ladybird, constructed through previous experiences and in consideration of desired responses, created a sense of unity among them.

The process of interpretive reproduction itself (Corsaro 2011) could also be read with a Bakhtinian lens. The potential of embedding Bakhtin's work on the dialogic, and humour and the carnivalesque (1968), to an analysis of children's interactions (with each other and adults) has been written about extensively by White (2009, 2011, 2014, 2015b, 2015a, 2021). Looking specifically at how mealtimes unfold in early years settings, White invites us to think of children's play and humour as key ways in which agency, resistance, reciprocity, and the continuous development of children's sense of self in relation to others is achieved (2014, 909). Similarly, Albon and Rosen have argued that Bakhtinian theory is useful to shed light on the dynamic relationship between the self and the other that children (and adults) engage in to create meaningful knowledge (2014, 9) in early years settings.

Thus, Bakhtin's work about speech acts and the dialogic can be deemed applicable to phenomenological conceptualisations of the self, both on a subjective and intersubjective level. Like the peer culture that emerged and developed during and through mealtimes, this circular process of becoming has a dual function; of resisting adults' attempts at control, but also of reproducing some of the mealtime norms and knowledge that adults deem valuable. This is exemplified by Alcock (2007), also in the context of the early years. Following Corsaro's work, she highlights the way by which toddlers in a childcare setting in New Zealand "re-create and adapt rules" through play behaviour by making new meanings, together, during what can often be unstimulating time spent eating at nursery (2007, 281–82). By integrating adult and children's perspectives about this activity, the author shows that just as there are differences between what children and adults want to achieve during mealtimes, there are also similarities. On the one hand, children overturned and contested pre-established patterns. On the other, they "[used] their imaginations to re-create and make internal sense of external (sociocultural) rules" (ibid., 282), ultimately repro-ducing one of the aims of the mealtime, which is to promote conviviality. Ultimately, however, the main purpose of mealtimes for the teachers was to provide nutritious meals, whilst for the children these were opportunities to create "playful together-ness" (ibid., 290). As I have argued throughout this chapter, at Ladybird adults were also usually concerned by *what* children ate, whereas what seemed to matter to chil-dren the most was *how* their mealtimes were carried out, and the ways in which they could interact with each other during these occasions. Unpacking this tension adds to the broader theme this book explores: *what* children eat fits into the universalism of policy, whereas *how* they eat can only be examined through the particularism of everyday caring relations. Applying Bakhtin's work on the dialogic to an exploration of care helps us to understand care as a relational category, one that relies on a back-and-forth exchange of words and practices that requires special attention.

Humour and the carnivalesque in early years settings

In addition to applying Bakhtin's work on the dialogic to the study of children's peer cultures, his work on humour and the carnivalesque (1968) has also been extremely influential to explore interactions within early years settings. Based on an analysis of French author Rabelais' writing, Bakhtin developed a theory that shows humour's role in overturning norms and power relations during the feasts and carnivals depicted in the authors' novels. In Bakhtin's own words:

> [The] temporary suspension…of hierarchical ranks created during carnival time a special type of communication impossible in everyday life. This led to the creation of special forms of…speech and gesture, frank and free, per-mitting no distance between those who came in contact with each other and liberating from norms of etiquette and decency imposed at other times.
>
> (1968, 10)

To Bakhtin, humour and laughter in the context of carnival is a clear defiance and resistance to power, and a space for the creation of new, shared meanings among those who contest authority (ibid., 16). The carnivalesque represents a moment when carnival participants – or players – indulge in a time of pleasure, role rever-sals, and crassness (Nolas, Varvantakis, and Aruldoss 2018, 11).

Playful and momentary transgressions of norms – like the blurring of hierarchical boundaries in Rabelais' carnival – are pervasive in children's peer groups. White (2014) provides a thorough account of how different scholars have applied this vision of resistance through humour to research in educational settings, including to the early years. Of particular note is her exploration of mealtimes in these contexts (2014, 2017). Like what I observed at Ladybird, White shows that mealtimes, as opposed to other daily events at the nursery she conducted research in, were moments of intense learning, and which were less child-led than most other activities (2017). Importantly, she notes that these acts of transgression would not be meaningful nor unifying for the children if adults did not embody an authoritative or disciplining role within the settings (2014, 908). Similarly, Nolas, Varvantakis, and Aruldoss (2018) have also noted that humour and role-play – as strategies children employ to subvert power relations – can also be understood through Bakhtin's work on the carnivalesque. Drawing from their own ethnography, they contend that humour helps children point to and create contradictions in their daily lives, and jokes and laughter feel particularly irreverent when met by adults' rejection and disapproval (2018, 12).

At Ladybird, humour provided children a channel through which to divert mealtime conversations away from adults' control, robbing the pedagogical element of these events from them. Often, children would make jokes about bodily processes to evoke humour and laughter in the peer group, which was deemed inappropriate by the staff:

For a couple of weeks now, the children's silverware has been missing from the children's centre, so we have had to use plastic cutlery at teaclub instead. This has not gone unnoticed by the children, and Crystal brings it up today as she struggles to stab a piece of broccoli with her plastic fork. A humorous conversation between Ruby and the children, about what could have possibly happened to the metal cutlery, ensues: "Is it in the microwave?" "Is it in the fridge?" "Maybe it's in Robert's office!" Fred [three-years-old] says, "I think Fran hid it!" I reply jokingly: "No, I wouldn't do that!" and he continues, "I think you hid it in the oven!" "In the oven?!" I say. "Yes," he says, "Or I think you pooped on them!" I tell him that, "I really wouldn't do that!" and he says, "Or maybe you just peed on them! Or farted on them!" I laugh and keep saying that I wouldn't do any of those things. I notice that Ruby has meanwhile stopped partaking in the conversation, and she soon stops us from continuing with these jokes: "This is not something we talk about at the table," she says, bringing the jokes to a stop – fieldnotes, April 2017.

Most provocations by children were engaged with and recognised by the staff: Joyce once told me I should research why children wave their cutlery around at the table, saying she thought it is because "*utensils are bigger than their hands and it makes them feel powerful.*" Similarly, Ruby's change of tone during the conversation about the missing cutlery signalled that talk of 'poo' and 'pee' were perceived as 'threats' or attempts by children to overtake adults' pedagogical roles at the table, which, in addition, can make the playful behaviour even more delightful and unifying for the children (Marjanovic-Shane and White 2014, 130). In this case, children's talk not only shifted the conversation about food and eating away from the control of adults, but it also challenged the much larger 'civilising' project, as described by Lupton and Fischler, that food and mealtimes are implicated in.

It is thus through children's engagement with each other, and the development of the self in relation to others, that peer cultures, with their own specific aims, can simultaneously oppose and reproduce facets of the adult world which they inhabit (as also shown in the discussion on the dialogic above). The degree to which this balance was achieved, I believe, depended on how much control adults exerted on children during mealtimes. Children who used extended hours services, for instance, had a lot more freedom and choice during mealtimes than they did at the nursery. As mentioned earlier in this chapter, children who attended breakfast club and tea-club were perceived by the staff to be "more independent" than the others. Joyce said this to me over the course of the first few weeks I spent at Ladybird, saying that the 'tea-clubbers' needed the least amount of help because "*they knew what to do*"; when they came in to the children's centre from the nursery they would independently hang their coats, go to the toilet if they needed to, wash their hands before sitting at the table, pour themselves drinks, and help each other (as well as discipline each other) during snack time and supper.

The nature of these interactions was not static, and I observed significant differences in how children behaved at these times depending on the staff member that assisted them. A certain approach could create a space for children that – although still largely controlled by adults – allowed them to express their preferences (within the limits of the foods available to them), and where they could overturn some of the mealtime norms and regulations. This was perceived as valuable by adults who emphasised the convivial aspect of meals. However, when food took on a pedagogical, as opposed to a convivial role, it was a lot more likely that children would not always react in ways that were considered acceptable by the adult running tea-club, as observed in the playful interaction described earlier, in which Fred joked about me 'pooping,' 'peeing,' or 'farting' on the missing cutlery, which elicited Ruby's disapproval. These moments shed useful insights about the limits of adults' involvement in shaping children's food practices, and the different ways in which children's agency and empowerment manifested themselves. Using Bakhtin's work on the dialogic and the carnivalesque emphasises the tension children try to navigate at nursey between *what* they eat and *how* they eat. The first fits within the universalism of policy, whilst the latter is revealed by examining the particularism of everyday caring relations.

Notes

1 A cereal brand.
2 This last motto was sometimes adopted by children to achieve the exact opposite of sharing. For instance, if someone wanted the last bit of something at the table they would invoke this saying to prevent others from having it.

3 The school staff believed Simon was on the autism spectrum, although a formal diagnosis had not been made yet at the time during which I conducted fieldwork.
4 Simon was not the only child I met that experienced this kind of problem during school meals; one other boy at the nursery, Theo (four-years-old), and a girl who was a regular attendee of the children's centre, Mimi (three), also had similar issues related to having been born prematurely.
5 Challenging each other to eat the most of something, to then be crowned the 'winner' at eating that particular food.
6 By placing the breadsticks underneath their upper lips so that they stuck out like fangs.
7 I did this gesture and called it 'vampire teeth' in an attempt to cheer up a boy called Adam one day at tea-club. This also offered a moment for me to reflect on in relation to doing research with children, and my aim of conducting an 'empathetic ethnography' (Clark 2010; Oakley 2015).

References

Albon, Deborah, and Rachel Rosen. 2014. *Negotiating Adult-Child Relationships in Early Childhood Research*. London: Routlegde.
Alcock, Sophie. 2007. 'Playing with Rules around Routines: Children Making Mealtimes Meaningful and Enjoyable'. *Early Years* 27 (3): 281–93. https://doi.org/10.1080/09575140701594426.
Bakhtin, Mikhail. 1968. *Rabelais and His World*. Cambridge, MA: MIT Press.
———. 1986. *Speech Genres and Other Late Essays*. Austin: University of Texas Press.
Clark, Alison. 2010. *Transforming Children's Spaces: Children's and Adults' Participation in Designing Learning Environments*. Abingdon: Routlegde.
Cohen, Lynn E. 2017. 'Preschool Discourse Interactions: Playful Meaning Making from a Carnival Lens'. *Knowledge Cultures* 5 (3): 60. https://doi.org/10.22381/KC5320175.
Corsaro, William. 2011. *The Sociology of Childhood*. London: SAGE Publications.
Elliott, Charlene. 2010. 'Eatertainment and the (Re)Classification of Children's Foods'. *Food, Culture & Society* 13 (4): 539–53. https://doi.org/10.2752/175174410X12777254289385.
Fischler, Claude. 1988. 'Food, Self and Identity'. *Social Science Information* 27 (2): 275–92.
———. 2011. 'Commensality, Society and Culture'. *Social Science Information* 50 (3–4): 28–548.
Flowers, Rick, and Elaine Swan. 2016. *Food Pedagogies*. London: Routledge.
Gardiner, Michael, and Michael Mayerfeld Bell. 1998. 'Bakhtin and the Human Sciences: A Brief Introduction'. In *Bakhtin and the Human Sciences: No Last Words*, edited by Michael Mayerfeld Bell and Michael Gardiner. London: SAGE Publications.
Goffman, Erving. 1968. *Asylums. Essays on the Social Situations of Mental Patients and Other Inmates* 1–12. New York: Anchor Books.
Lupton, Deborah. 1996. *Food, the Body and the Self*. London: SAGE Publications.
Mandell, Nancy. 1988. 'The Least-Adult Role in Studying Children.' Journal of Contemporary Ethnography, 16(4), 433–467. https://doi.org/10.1177/0891241688164002
Marjanovic-Shane, Ana, and E. Jayne White. 2014. 'When the Footlights Are Off: A Bakhtinian Interrogation of Play as Postupok'. *International Journal of Play* 3 (2): 119–35. https://doi.org/10.1080/21594937.2014.931686.
Nolas, Sevasti-Melissa, Vinnarasan Aruldoss, and Christos Varvantakis. 2018. 'Learning to Listen: Exploring the Idioms of Childhood'. *Sociological Research Online*, 24(3), 1–20.
Nolas, Sevasti-Melissa, Christos Varvantakis, and Vinnarasan Aruldoss. 2017. 'Talking Politics in Everyday Family Lives'. *Contemporary Social Science* 12 (1–2): 68–83. https://doi.org/10.1080/21582041.2017.1330965.
Oakley, Ann. 2015. 'Interviewing Women Again: Power, Time and the Gift'. Sociology, 1–19.

Tallant, Laura. 2015. 'Framing Young Children's Humour and Practitioner Responses to It Using a Bakhtinian Carnivalesque Lens'. *International Journal of Early Childhood* 47 (2): 251–66. https://doi.org/10.1007/s13158-015-0134-0.

———. 2017. 'Embracing the Carnivalesque: Young Children's Humour as Performance and Communication'. *Knowledge Cultures* 5 (3): 71. https://doi.org/10.22381/KC5320176.

Tobin, Joseph, Yen Hsueh, and Mayumi Karasawa. 2009. *Preschool in Three Cultures Revisited: China, Japan, and the United States*. Chicago: The University of Chicago Press.

Warming, Hanne. 2005. 'Participant Observation: A Way to Learn about Children's Perspectives'. In *Beyond Listening: Children's Perspectives on Early Childhood Services*, edited by Alison Clark, Anne-Trine Kjørholt, and Peter Moss, 51–70. Bristol: The Policy Press.

White, E. Jayne. 2009. 'A Bakhtinian Homecoming: Operationalizing Dialogism in the Context of an Early Childhood Education Centre in Wellington, New Zealand'. *Journal of Early Childhood Research* 7 (3): 299–323. https://doi.org/10.1177/1476718X09336972.

———. 2011. 'Response to the School of the Dialogue of Cultures as a Dialogic Pedagogy'. *Journal of Russian & East European Psychology* 49 (2): 77–82. https://doi.org/10.2753/RPO1061-0405490212.

———. 2015a. 'Bringing Dialogism to Bear in the Early Years'. *International Journal of Early Childhood* 47 (2): 213–16. https://doi.org/10.1007/s13158-015-0145-x.

———. 2015b. 'Who Is Bakhtin?' *International Journal of Early Childhood* 47 (2): 217–19. https://doi.org/10.1007/s13158-015-0144-y.

———. 2017. 'A Feast of Fools: Mealtimes as Democratic Acts of Resistance and Collusion in Early Childhood Education'. *Knowledge Cultures* 5 (3): 85. https://doi.org/10.22381/KC5320177.

———. 2021. 'Mikhail Bakhtin: A Two-Faced Encounter with Child Becoming(s) through Dialogue'. *Early Child Development and Care* 191 (7–8): 1277–86. https://doi.org/10.1080/03004430.2020.1840371.

White, Elizabeth Jayne. 2014. 'Are You "Avin a Laff?": A Pedagogical Response to Bakhtinian Carnivalesque in Early Childhood Education'. *Educational Philosophy and Theory* 46 (8): 898–913. https://doi.org/10.1080/00131857.2013.781497.

5 Food and parenting in the mixed economy of welfare

In Chapter 1, I used Bacchi and Goodwin's 'What's the Problem Represented to be?' (WPR) approach (2016) to examine how 'problems' related to children's diets are framed in official discourse (i.e. as a consequence of 'bad' parenting, lack of knowledge/skills, and insufficient early intervention) predominantly by examining secondary sources. This chapter now turns to exploring how these framings of the 'problems' have had an impact within the wider context of the borough where I conducted research. I will predominantly focus on the interactions that took place during a series of cooking courses delivered at Ladybird Nursery and Children's Centre by a local charity that I have renamed 'Green Kitchen.' This case study will be central to the chapter, yet I will also focus on two other interventions aimed at 'target parents': the Rose Voucher scheme and Health, Exercise and Nutrition for the Really Young, or HENRY (also analysed using the WPR approach in Chapter 1). As I will show, parallels can be drawn in how each initiative was promoted in the community as well as the aims and outcomes that were sought through these interventions.

To examine how different national and local moral discourses about food were negotiated on the ground through these interventions, I will analyse data collected during Green Kitchen sessions during the preliminary fieldwork stage in January and March 2016, as well as during a six-week long course the organisation delivered in March 2017. Thus, the purpose of this chapter is to empirically assess how the official discourses that I unpacked earlier in this book unfold in the lives of 'target groups,' and how the assumptions underlying these discourses shape the interactions between those who promote interventions and the families that are recruited to take part in them.

Simultaneously, this chapter also offers an account of how services in the Mixed Economy of Welfare (henceforth MEW) operate using a Foucauldian lens. I argue that 'knowledge' and 'expertise' are a fundamental way by which governmentality is enacted within this welfare model and the interventions within it. Linking this framework to discourses and interventions which rest on the assumption that individual choice is a key determinant of health outcomes, I will show that the structural barriers that prevent people from accessing nutritious food are often ignored. Viewing the matter instead as an issue of people's lack of knowledge, information and/or skills, can fall short.

DOI: 10.4324/9781003297642-6

Thus, exploring the contradictions and arbitrariness inherent in food and family interventions brings the challenges that parents face when feeding their children to the fore, again pointing to the incompatibility of policy's universalism with the particularism of caring through food.

The 'wrong kind of parent'

Yesterday, Elsa [Ladybird's community outreach coordinator] asked Kate [early years practitioner] whether she can help her to do some community outreach work with her, as there have been no parents signing up for a vegan cooking course (provided by a local community kitchen initiative, 'Green Kitchen') that begins next week at the children's centre. I ask them if I can join them in this task; after getting Robert's [Ladybird's extended services manager] approval, I join Elsa and Kate at 9.30 a.m. and we set off, clipboards, posters, and leaflets in hand.

The plan is to visit the different housing estates near the children's centre, to reach out to 'target families' with children under five years old. Elsa and Kate don't have a specific strategy to go about this, and Elsa says we also have to be careful where we leave the information since we "could get into trouble" if we leave it in common areas or hang it on walls. On the way to the first estate, Elsa says that it has taken a while to build a connection with the person in charge of this estate's community outreach work, so that we really should be careful, that it is important "not to break the contact" because this person has all the information they need to take their own community outreach strategy forward.

We get to the first block in the housing estate, and Kate knows that the main door will open by pressing the button marked 'Provider' on the buzzer (this is the case within a margin of a few hours each morning, so that the postman can enter to leave the mail, she says). We don't know how to proceed after we go in; Kate decides to leave some leaflets on the steps of the main stairwell.

When we arrive to the second estate, Elsa rings the doorbell to one of the ground floor flats; a woman that she knows (and is registered at the children's centre) opens the door, and her young son, a toddler of about two, appears behind her to greet us. The woman seems happy to see Elsa and Kate. After a brief catch up, Elsa explains that we are sharing information about the cooking course; after sharing a leaflet with her, she asks her if she knows any other families with children under five years old living in her estate. The woman mentions a couple of flat numbers and we go into the block to slide leaflets under those flats' doors.

On the way out, we bump into another woman and her son; she is also known to the staff at the children's centre, and I remember seeing her on several occasions. Elsa and Kate tell her what we are doing, and she seems interested in the cooking course. After reading the leaflet that Kate gives her, she regretfully says she can't make it because she signed her son up for swimming lessons on Wednesdays at 11am (same time as the cooking course). She offers to take some leaflets to give to other parents that she knows in her building. Once she is gone, Elsa laments quietly that she was "the wrong kind of parent" to whom to promote the cooking classes to...

As we walk to the next place, I ask Elsa a few questions about the 'target families,' and how they know who they are. She tells me that each year the children's centre needs to meet a certain goal of 'target families' to reach and include in their activities, and that their funding from the council depends partly on reaching this objective. She tells me that "The [education authority] is really on it," so it's important that they meet their outcomes. I ask her what kind of families they need to involve in the initiatives. She says it's "mainly white working class families with boys, Afro-Caribbean families, Turkish families, and families with any members that are out of employment." I ask her how they access this information, and she says the council shares this with them, although the council accesses this data from the NHS.

We arbitrarily slide flyers under every other door in the next housing estate we visit, and then we move on to the nearby health centre, where we meet another woman that Elsa and Kate know, with her baby. They persuade her to sign up to the course, so she writes her name down on the form (becoming the first participant on the list). As we exit the building, they share information about the course with another woman who is by the entrance with her baby: she does not sign up.

The next stop is a children's centre, where we leave some flyers with the staff members. Elsa seemed uncomfortable about advertising for the cooking course there. She tells me that this children's centre (as others in the area) are "competitors" for funding, but she also wonders about this centre's future: "I don't know how long they can keep open." Indeed, I notice that this children's centre is much smaller than the one at Ladybird, and seems quite rundown by comparison.

The final stop is the nearby park, where we meet another mother who is registered at Ladybird's children's centre; she is playing with her son and new-born child at the playground. We share information about the cooking course and she agrees to sign up. We see another boy we know from the children's centre playing at the park with his grandfather, who the woman we are talking to also knows. As they approach us, the woman mentions the course to the grandfather, and asks him if he thinks the boy's mother would be interested in taking part. They decide to call her and ask if she would like to join. After hanging up, she writes both her and the other woman's names on the sign-up sheet – fieldnotes, February 2017.

This instance stood out, and still stands out, as one of the most emblematic from my year of fieldwork. It shows the ways in which policy-level initiatives and assumptions play out in practice in the everyday lives of the people I worked with, both the practitioners and the families. It reflects some of the (sometimes) erratic techniques that actors engaging in policy initiatives follow in the pursuit of seemingly 'rational' bureaucratic goals (e.g. Gupta 2012) – Elsa and Kate's informal community outreach strategy supported one of Ladybird's key organisational objectives. It highlights that food, morality, and parenting are deeply interlinked, helping me to think about other similar situations I encountered during my time doing research, and about the experiences that participants shared with me. Further, this episode provided a powerful insight into how MEW (Powell 2014) functions in practice, and how its different components (public, charitable, private) intersect.

MEW in Britain is composed by state, market, voluntary, and informal (i.e. family and friends) welfare provision (Powell 2014, 2). This fragmentation in the provision of welfare services follows the core principles of advanced liberalism, where the political and ethical rationales that (should) underpin welfare provision are separated from the management and delivery of services (Stewart and Walsh 1992, 506). Within this model, ever increasing numbers of services and providers are wanted, yet all must follow the same standards of efficiency, 'value for money,' and measurable results (Moss and Petrie 2000, 74). This political context, paired with the entrenchment of 'audit culture' (Rose 1996, 55; Power 1999; Shore 2017) in both the public and private sectors, has led to service fragmentation, and to what Gupta (2012) has described as the arbitrary results of welfare policies, which often (paradoxically) perpetuate and uphold the structural inequalities that policy seeks to redress (2012, 31). Gupta contends, however, that this is not so much a consequence of official actors' indifference or lack of motivation, but a result of the bureaucratic system within which they work (ibid., 23).

Elsa's comment about the 'wrong kind of parent' in the ethnographic vignette above is a poignant and unintentional contradiction. The woman she labelled this way was considered one of the "posh mummies" by some of the early years practitioners at Ladybird, a term they sometimes used to refer to middle-class parents, often white British. The comment seemed contradictory to me, because the service being promoted was intended for parents whose skills and practices are often perceived as deficient, in need of improvement. The middle-class mother was the 'wrong kind of parent' to whom Green Kitchen's cooking course should be promoted, because she was assumed to be the 'right kind of parent' in a more general sense, one whose parenting skills were assumed to be adequate. Elsa's comment thus reflected a more widely and long-held notion in England, both in policy and mainstream discourse, about which parents are in need of policy interventions, and which are not.[1]

The approach that Ladybird followed to promote the cooking classes also says something about the bureaucratic and policy context within which most state-maintained early years settings in the U.K. operate. As Elsa explained to me, targeted family interventions (with specific outcomes and objectives to be met) need to be promoted and implemented to ensure that funding will continue to be provided to the children's centre.

'Good food,' 'healthy choices,' and the individualisation of health

Policy discourses mediate power relations between those who are the authoritative voices in any given 'policy community' (Eisenberg 2011) and those at whom policies are directed. Bacchi and Goodwin propose that understanding the tensions that emerge from those relationships is a fruitful way to examine power and resistance (2016, 31), borrowing from Foucault's famous conjecture that there cannot be power without resistance (1978).

Parents targeted for interventions were by no means passive when engaging with Ladybird staff members and other official and non-official actors in the community, as will be shown. Nonetheless, in this context it is important to think about who determined what 'good food' is, both on a macro- and micro-level, and how expertise and authority were construed and enacted by different people. Expertise and knowledge are important categories to examine; those who are positioned (or position themselves) as experts tend to accumulate a level of power that is often difficult to challenge (Rose 1996, 50). Therefore the notion of *savoir*, or knowledge (Foucault 1991, 100), is also important to this analysis. According to Procacci, the function of *savoir* is to position ideas and people within specific sets of relationships, so that 'scientifically backed' interventions can be justified when being implemented (1991, 156–57). This is what Lupton also suggests when arguing that "Public health and health promotion depend on knowledges to effect governmentality" (1995, 49).

Examining how discourses about food and nutrition were used in the family interventions that I observed at Ladybird revealed how expertise and authority hold power. To families, food's goodness also includes the pleasurable, social, and caring dimension of feeding and eating (e.g. Albon 2005; Harman, Faircloth, and Cappellini 2019), not just the more biomedical understanding of what 'healthy food' is. Yet, public health standards often undermined, or outright excluded, what parents might think constitutes 'good food.' Policy 'problems' to be solved via interventions are also framed within a number of specific knowledges (Lupton 1995; Bacchi 2010; Bacchi and Goodwin 2016). Lee contends, for example, that an overlap between policy domains (public health and family intervention) has fuelled moral claims about parenting practices, which are judged against the 'health behaviours' that parents follow and/or promote to their children (2011, 4). Parents' feeding practices are thus subject to scrutiny, not only from official actors, but also each other and themselves, as I will show.

Following Bacchi and Goodwin's "What's the Problem Represented to be?" (WPR) approach (2016), and Mosse's (2005) and Gupta's (2012) work on policy, in Chapter 1 I argued that public health and family intervention policy models still rest on the assumption that access to services that provide information and/ or training to users will lead to behaviour change. I have also argued that an emphasis on individual accountability (i.e. assuming that society is populated by 'self-governing' individuals) as a determinant of health outcomes is characteristic of Britain's advanced liberal context. By extension, current policy paradigms here tend to rest on the assumption that there are technical solutions for every 'problem,' a range of mechanisms with which to achieve specific outcomes (Rose 1996, 57). Drawing from Rose (1999), Moss and Petrie critique this 'managerialist' approach in British policymaking, claiming that it promotes a positivist vision which "promises rationalised order and certainty, removing politics and ethics and replacing them with techniques of control" (2000, 76). This, in turn, contributes to the fragmentation of welfare services (see, e.g. Randall 2000) leading to a more market-oriented model of both supplying and accessing provisions.

Drawing from Gupta's work (2012), what is interesting about this fragmentation (paired with the underlying assumption that policy frameworks are neutral and rational) are the arbitrary results that many policy initiatives have, and the seemingly unchanging approaches to applying them. This is particularly so for public health interventions around food and eating. There is ample literature suggesting that the evidence on the effectiveness of interventions that are nutrition-driven, market-based, and rest on the notion of individual accountability for behavioural change, can be patchy and contradictory (see, e.g. Cummins 2005; Caraher and Dowler 2007; Betty 2013; Evans 2017; Wake 2018). With particular emphasis on the issue of food poverty, some scholars have proposed that a rights-based approach to food policy is necessary to shed light on the structural, rather than individual, factors that have an impact on health outcomes, and call to increase state responsibility to ensure equal access to food (e.g. Dowler 2002; Chilton and Rose 2009; Lang and Rayner 2010; Lang 2019). As Dowler and O'Connor have argued for the British and Irish cases, states have repeatedly failed to recognise that enforcing mechanisms such as social benefits or minimum wage policies will not guarantee people's access to sufficient and adequate food, and this is especially the case for families with children (2012, 48). As many scholars continue to show, the most significant proportion of households in the U.K. with children living in relative poverty have at least one working adult living in them (O'Connell, Knight, and Brannen 2019, 9), although families where parents are unemployed or underemployed are the most at risk of poverty and food insecurity (Brannen and O'Connell 2022, 2).

Governments' inabilty to fully protect households' right to food is also a consequence of the fragmentation caused by MEW, where state responsibility to ensure access to essential services is transferred to non-governmental bodies and civil society. Family interventions such as the ones I will explore in this chapter can be thus understood in line with the definition of MEW, as pertaining to the voluntary component of welfare services provision in Britain. Alcott and Scott analyse the rise of the voluntary sector as complementary to, and overlapping with, both state and market services, as well as being an important avenue for civil society to take action on social justice matters (2014, 84). With this plethora of competing actors, all working with their own sets of assumptions, goals, approaches, and constraints to reach similar goals, come inconsistent and transient policy results. Exploring the contradictions and arbitrariness inherent in food and family interventions can help reveal the challenges that parents face when feeding their children, which often have little to do with a lack of knowledge about nutrition or cooking skills. Doing so also sheds further light on the incompatibility of policy's universalism with the particularism of caring through food, which this book seeks to unpack.

Green Kitchen and the borough

Green Kitchen is a local community kitchen project, founded in 2011. On their website, their "food policy" involves promoting 'healthier diets' through four key guiding principles: local, organic, seasonal, and plant-based (vegan). The organisation runs as a charity, financed by a number of local and national donors. They also charge for providing courses to schools and community centres, organising bespoke events, hiring out their headquarters' kitchen to groups, and conducting consultancy work. The borough's cultural and ethnic diversity is also acknowledged on their website, where they assert their commitment to address the rise of non-communicable diseases like type 2 diabetes (particularly among disadvantaged groups), and to promote inclusion in the community.

Green Kitchen delivered three, six-week-long vegan cooking courses to families registered at Ladybird's children's centre over the time I spent carrying out my research. Ten places were available for each course, although attendance was often patchy. The classes were advertised to mothers and fathers alike, nonetheless all the attendees that I met were women. Unlike some of the other workshops offered at the children's centre, such as candle-making or cupcake decoration, parents could bring their children with them to the cooking classes, and children were encouraged to also get involved with the preparation of the meals.

Each class ran over a two-hour and half period, and was delivered by a chef employed by Green Kitchen and a volunteer assistant. Each course was run by a different chef: Clare, Andy, and Judith, and each of them had a volunteer working with them. None of the women I met were professionally trained as chefs – they were all self-taught, and had years of experience cooking and teaching cookery classes. Volunteers, like the chefs, were also driven to join the organisation because of their personal interest in food and health. Anna, the volunteer working with Judith, had also recently completed a degree in nutritional science, which she put to use during the educational component of the course she helped deliver. At the end of each class, the families, Ladybird staff, and members of Green Kitchen would come together to eat the meal that they had prepared.[2]

Classes were structured around preparing two or three recipes (usually a main and two sides, or a main, a side, and a dessert). At the beginning of each class, the chef and volunteer distributed chopping boards, plastic knives,[3] and ingredients on the small tables in the main room of the children's centre, around which the parents (and, intermittently, the children) would sit around in a convivial manner for the duration of the session. Tasks were carried out in a kind of assembly line, with everyone getting a different ingredient ready to make the recipes, which were then cooked by the chefs and volunteers in the kitchen within the children's centre. Conversation would run freely as parents and Ladybird staff chopped herbs and vegetables, putting them into bowls before being incorporated into the meal being prepared. Occasionally, parents would be invited into the kitchen to observe the chef while she cooked, or help her stir the food while she attended to other kitchen duties. Parents thus did not actively partake in the cooking but were very much involved in the preparation of the meals.

The sessions also included more formal educational components, often about healthy eating in general, as well as the benefits of adopting a plant-based diet. This aspect of the courses also provided a deeper insight into the rationale of Green Kitchen chefs and volunteers. The didactic element of the sessions was implemented less formally in the first two courses I observed, whereas in subsequent sessions the volunteer assistant delivered brief lecture-style talks half-way through the sessions (usually whilst the main dish was cooking), during which she addressed different topics about food and diet, and parents were given materials[4] to carry out activities related to these after each talk.

Although public health messaging played a central role in the classes, the service was deliberately not advertised as a 'healthy cooking' course to families. When I asked Joyce (the lead early years practitioner at the children's centre) why this was the case, she told me that it was already difficult to encourage parents to take part in this activity, and advertising it as a healthy cooking course would only deter them further. Joyce's remark was striking; first, it reflected the often-held and paternalistic assumption that 'target groups' are being intervened upon without their knowledge. Second, implicit in this statement is also a recognition that people generally do not want to be told how to change their 'health behaviours,' as pointed out in some of the critiques of public health interventions cited above. Further, this instance showed how the overlap between public health and family policy also blurs the aims of these interventions, so it is important to ask whether improving eating or improving 'parenting styles' took precedence in this context.

Official discourses about food and nutrition were prevalent in the interactions between Green Kitchen's staff and the parents that attended the cooking classes. Although veganism was by no means portrayed as representative of official discourses, Green Kitchen co-opted these messages in their own narrative about healthy eating.[5] Creating an awareness about 'healthy eating,' as well as the benefits of adopting a more plant-based diet, were central components of the sessions.

Green Kitchen's adherence to a vegan philosophy should also be contextualised in line with recent changes happening within a borough that is becoming increasingly gentrified. As in many other parts of the U.K., and London in particular, the arrival of young middle and upper-middle class professionals to the area has led to an exponential rise in housing and other living costs, displacing local communities and businesses (Wessendorf 2014, 107). Veganism, in this context, can signify an important class marker, whether it be representative of individuals' financial or cultural capital, if not both, and this is the angle that this chapter seeks to explore. Of course, generalisations about the vegan movement need to be considered carefully. As Harper argues, "the culture of veganism itself is comprised of many different subcultures and philosophies" (in Alkon and Agyeman 2011, 222), also including different religious and spiritual practices.

However, as will be further explored below, in a context of socio-economic disparity, and within a heavily industrialised food system such as London's, the cost and practicalities of being vegan and buying organic food, as they were presented to the parents that took part in the courses, seemed to pose some contradictions that were either ignored or dismissed by Green Kitchen members. Further, given that the children's centre was facing funding cuts, the fact that Ladybird paid Green Kitchen a significant amount of money for each course delivered can also be problematised, and is in line with some of the critiques about the 'competitive tendering' of services that has emerged within MEW (Stewart and Walsh 1992; Moss and Petrie 2000). By treating veganism as a class marker in this chapter, I also aim to show how this practice became a vehicle through which expertise and *savoir* were operationalised.

Another critique levelled at food advocacy groups is the 'educational' approach they can often follow, with an aim both to improve people's health but also address ethical matters (such as animal welfare or climate change). Writing in the context of the United States, Guthman contends that alternative food movements generally tend to perceive lack of knowledge as the key barrier to achieving a healthier, more ethical food system, as opposed to structural issues (Guthman, Julie 2011, 263; see also Semple 2022, 94). Focusing on race relations in particular, Guthman further argues that one of the reasons these initiatives might not be successful in diverse and/or disadvantaged communities is because the language and practices they operate under are exclusionary (ibid., 275).

"It's better because it's plant based": vegan morality and individual accountability

During the first two cooking courses that I observed, certain tensions arose that indicate how the moral dimensions of food, parenting, and class intersect in daily life – as they also tend to do in official and mainstream discourse. These tensions also reflect the broader history of children's centres as sites within which official actors and early years practitioners offer 'training' to 'target families' (Macvarish in Lee et al. 2014, 90–91). Focusing on the direction of knowledge flows during these classes, for instance, which was largely top-down and unidirectional, reveals some of the assumptions Green Kitchen chefs and volunteers made about the parents they interacted with. It also highlights the need to examine discourses about food and diet through the lens of power, and how these translate into practice (Baez and Talburt 2008; Maher, Fraser, and Lindsay 2010; Maher, Fraser, and Wright 2010; Morris and Featherstone 2010).

The NHS and Public Health England recommendations (particularly those around salt and sugar avoidance) were dominant in many of the interactions I observed during Green Kitchen's lessons. One day in January, Clare, the chef, invited two women into the kitchen to stir a pasta sauce that was simmering on the hob. The two participants were migrants from East Africa, and had expressed their enthusiasm for food and cooking during the Green Kitchen sessions, often talking about the dishes they prepared at home and their eagerness for their young daughters to start trying spicier meals as they grew older. When invited into the kitchen that day, they tasted the sauce and asked Clare if she would add any salt to it, to which Clare responded:

> *Salt? You use salt in your cooking? You give salt to your children? Salt is bad for you, and every time you use it your children become used to the taste and they'll always want more. Why do you want to put salt in here when we have all these lovely spices?*

During the sessions she ran, Clare did not conceal her personal views about food and eating, which were enmeshed in the principles promoted by Green Kitchen and public health messaging. Some of her comments were also telling about the reasons she believed that people did not cook from scratch or used ingredients she deemed inadequate, like canned beans. On several occasions, she insisted that using canned beans or legumes instead of buying the dry equivalent of these and soaking them overnight was a sign of laziness.

Tensions between parents and Green Kitchen chefs and volunteers, and among parents, rose to the surface as instances like these repeated themselves each week. This was particularly evident during a class that Andy, another Green Kitchen chef, ran. Although not as outspoken about her views, Andy also seemed to share some of Clare's preconceptions about the parents who attended the lessons, explaining she preferred to teach people how to make raw recipes, *"because people can be lazy or not make time to cook."*

It was most evident in Andy's classes how the moral dimensions of food, parenting, and class intersect. The group Andy taught was not only comprised of 'target parents,' but a more diverse group of participants. Intentionally or not, Andy predominantly invited those perceived as "posh mummies" into the kitchen to help her, on the rare occasions on which the stove was being used. I observed the same pattern when she distributed tasks to the group, often assigning simpler jobs (such as cutting up vegetables or herbs) to the 'target parents,' inadvertently revealing an assumption that they might be less skilled. Two of the participants complained about this (seemingly unintended) preferential treatment on a day in which we prepared pizza, and only three out of the eight mothers attending were asked to knead the dough, whilst the others were asked to chop the pizza toppings, a comparatively easier task.

Similarly, on this day when we made pizza, Andy and her volunteer assistant mistakenly did not bring the sufficient amount of ingredients needed to make enough salad for everyone, and when the time came for them to serve and distribute plates with food to the families, they seemed to prioritise giving the salad to the "posh mummies" and their children. This, again, led some parents to complain that they were not being treated fairly, which put Andy and the volunteer in an uncomfortable situation that they did not seem to anticipate. After the session ended, Andy approached me and shared her thoughts about what had happened during the session, commenting that she had not expected all the parents to be interested in trying the salad. This view seemed close to some of the stereotypes and assumptions that play into moral discourses about food and class in the U.K. (for an analysis of classed assumptions of Australian mothers' feeding practices see Maher, Fraser, and Wright 2010; for a discussion on the 'social value' of organic food see Costa, Zepeda, and Sirieix 2014).

Aside from these moments of tension, it was also the case that not all parents were persuaded by Green Kitchen's approach, philosophy, and methods. In particular, they often questioned their advocacy of plant-based diets, which some of the chefs and volunteers did not seem to expect. For example, one day when Andy shared a recipe to make a smoothie, she advised to substitute honey with date syrup to sweeten the drink, justifying this by saying that honey has a high sugar content so should be avoided. When one of the participants read the label on the bottle of date syrup, she noted that the sugar content in it was also quite high, and asked Andy why it was considered healthier than honey if it seemed to be just as sweet. When confronted, Andy simply responded, "*It's better because it's plant-based.*"

Preference for certain foods was also a factor that seemed to add to participants' (and some Ladybird staff's) scepticism towards Green Kitchen's vegan principles, as well as what they believed their children liked. Susan, a young single mother with a two-year-old son, once expressed that she was worried about her son not getting enough nutrients because he was a 'fussy eater' – a concern, as I showed in Chapter 3, that was prevalent among many parents and staff at Ladybird. She added that some of the things he really enjoyed eating (and ate more of) were chicken and milk, so she would never consider not feeding him these. Several parents and Ladybird staff admitted to simply liking the taste of meat, and on that basis they also did not express particular interest in transitioning to a plant-based diet.

The cost of food, however, was also a factor. Green Kitchen's website, and the chefs and volunteers I interacted with, emphasised that having a vegan diet and buying organic products is 'cheap.' Yet, they delivered conflicting messages on where to access cheap ingredients, at times referring to the local community gardens their organisation collaborated with, or nearby local markets – where fruits and vegetables do tend to be cheaper – but at other times referring to organic food shops, which can often be much more expensive. The insistence that having a plant-based diet is not costly seemed problematic, particularly due to the continuous rise in the cost of living that the U.K. has experienced since the Brexit referendum. Many scholars have voiced concern about the impact of high and fluctuating food prices in the U.K., particularly for those households in which food purchases represent a greater proportion of their expenditure (Ashton, Middleton, and Lang 2014; Jones et al. 2014; O'Connell et al. 2018; Lang 2019). In January 2017, the U.K. charity Food Ethics Council warned about "the beginning of the end of cheap food," releasing a report warning about the likely increment of food prices post-Brexit (Food Ethics Council 2017, 6). This is also particularly problematic given that, "The country's poorest households are already spending 20% of their incomes on food […] Arguably this encourages many households on low incomes to buy 'empty calorie' food rather than high quality fresh ingredients" (ibid., 7). At the time this book is being written, in mid-2023, these issues have only become more deeply entrenched as the cost of living crisis continues to curtail people's access to adequate nutrition (Goodwin 2022).

Missing from these discussions is also the fact that making 'cheap food' requires investment of other resources. Financial cost aside, some of the Green Kitchen recipes were time consuming and needed advanced planning (such as having to soak beans overnight or procure a lengthy list of ingredients), implied fuel costs, and required the use of kitchen utensils that not everyone has access to. It was also unclear what were the chefs' and volunteers' reference points for the prices of ingredients. Some encouraged participants to peruse their local corner stores or organic shops (which can be two rather different kinds of commercial settings, both in terms of price and available products), or one of their partner charity organisations, which ran a local community garden project from which fresh produce could be purchased. The ingredient lists for the recipes provided were often also rather long and required the purchase – or assumed people had – a long list of store cupboard staples that those who live hand to mouth are unlikely to have available.

A final domain to explore is the discourse of individual choice and accountability – also explored in Chapters 1 and 2 – that Green Kitchen adopted. This was particularly emphasised during the final course I observed, during which Anna, the volunteer assistant, led discussions about specific topics on health and nutrition during each class. One week, the subject covered was that of reading ingredient lists and labels on food packaging:

Anna says there are three different labels we need to pay attention to on packages: the ingredients list, the nutrition label, and the label in the front with the red, yellow, and green bubbles showing required daily intakes. She says that on the ingredient list, the first ingredient listed is usually the main ingredient, and that we should be careful about eating products with ingredient lists that are too long. With regards to sugar, she says that it has a lot of different names (dextrose, fructose, sacarose, any kind of syrup) so we should pay particular attention to those too. Paulette [one of the participants] says she's always careful with this because her eldest son, who is 13, has ADHD so he needs to avoid sugary foods (I thought this was an interesting comment showing a parent's own expert knowledge, but her contribution seems to go unnoticed). With regards to the red, yellow, and green labels, Anna mentions, as an example, that if we eat a particular food item containing 50% of the daily sugar intake then we really need to be careful about eating other sugary foods. She says that foods that have lots of red bubbles should really be only considered treats. The chat ends with an exercise involving cards with photos of food products in the front and the food labels and ingredients list in the back. She picks two cards and asks us to discuss which of the two are healthier – one shows a vegan brand snack bar, the other is a more commercial brand snack bar. Participants unanimously pick the vegan bar as the least healthy, because it contains a higher percentage of sugar; however Anna corrects them, because although the non-vegan option contains less sugar, it has a longer ingredients list, which she says is less healthy – fieldnotes, March 2017.

This interaction echoes Andy's statement that 'vegan is better,' further emphasising some of the contradictions already discussed, as well as showing again the top-down knowledge flow (from Green Kitchen to parents) in the cooking sessions. During Anna's talks, the public health approach that prioritises enhancing awareness and increasing knowledge about nutrition was prevalent, despite participants' prior knowledge, as shown by Paulette's comment in the above vignette.

Teaching people how to read food labels also fits with the market-based assumption that consumers are individually willing and able to, and responsible for, under-standing dietary information and making decisions based on this (Ulijaszek and McLennan 2016, 407), without taking into account the many constraints (financial and otherwise) that people face when purchasing and consuming food. When faced with contradictory messages about what 'good food' is (such as in this case), the problem is exacerbated. In this regard, Green Kitchen's activity also fits in the model of MEW already described, not only in terms of the service provision but also in its messaging, which combines elements from both the public sector and the food industry. In this way, an alternative food movement such as veganism, which purports to improve people's health and address the problems intrinsic to a deeply flawed food system, has also been co-opted by the rhetoric of the policy discourses I have critiqued throughout this book. To assume a position of expertise and authority – indeed, of power – Green Kitchen members followed the status quo promoted by policy and mainstream discourse, yet also presented themselves as an alternative to the status quo and as attempting to address structural issues. Again, this shows that individuals, organisations, and policymakers who occupy positions of authority create their expertise far removed from the contexts in which they operate, failing to address material and structural issues. This, in turn, can also delegitimise their role as experts.

Challenging policy assumptions: knowledge and skills vs. structural issues

The Rose Voucher scheme

> *I think people look at me and probably think I don't know how to cook and that I probably feed [my daughter]... Iceland[6] food... like freezer food all day – Louise, in a semi-structured interview, March 2017.*

Louise was one of the participants in Green Kitchen's cooking courses. She was one of the youngest mothers that I met at the children's centre – 20 at the time of our interview. She had a daughter who was one year and a half, and was an enthu-siastic member of the community. Being a single mother, out of employment, and living in temporary accommodation, she relied on welfare benefits – indeed, by these standards, she fit the description of the 'target parent' with whom Elsa and Kate wanted to engage, and her account above shows that she was fully aware that this is how she was perceived. Louise was also one of the most skilled and eager cooks among the parents I met during my fieldwork, and a talented baker. She pursued her culinary interests beyond Ladybird, first joining community baking and cake decoration courses, and eventually being accepted on an apprenticeship at a local bakery, which ran as a social enterprise. Therefore, and contrary to what might be assumed by her socio-economic status, Louise should not have been considered a 'target parent'[7] for an intervention on food and cooking given her knowledge and abilities.

Despite her level of knowledge and skill, she faced multiple challenges when cooking in the domestic sphere. Louise described how difficult it could be to make Emma (her daughter) the food that she deemed healthy and nutritious, due to the limited facilities in the hostel that she and Emma had been living in for over a year. She told me about their restricted fridge space and lack of freezer, and the challenges that can often arise when sharing a living space with strangers. For example, she told me she had more than once found the plastic containers she used to store their food melting on the electric hob in the shared kitchen facilities, an unpleasant prank she believed another resident of the hostel was playing on them. Aside from the restrictions that their living circumstances posed, her financial situation was also a challenge. During our interview, we spoke about the Rose Voucher scheme, which she made use of to acquire fresh fruits and vegetables from one of the local markets.

Elsa, in her capacity as community outreach coordinator, was also in charge of running the Rose Voucher scheme at Ladybird and other children's centres in the borough. The scheme is supported by the London-based Alexandra Rose Charity, founded in 1912 to aid Londoners living in poverty. Since 2014, the charity has directed its efforts increasingly towards projects aimed at tackling food poverty (Alexandra Rose Charity 2018b).

At the time of my research, the vouchers were being distributed across London, Liverpool, and Barnsley to families who are also eligible for Healthy Start[8] vouchers; "A family receives £3 of Rose Vouchers for each child, every week, or £6 if the child is under one years old" (Alexandra Rose Charity 2018a). The vouchers could be exclusively exchanged at stalls in local markets. In a semi-structured interview, Elsa explained to me that the programme began initially as a pilot scheme in November 2013, targeting 20 families within the borough where Ladybird was located. At the time of our interview in November 2016, 80 families in four different children's centres were involved, and Elsa considered the intervention largely successful. She told me that the comments she had received from parents in a recent evaluation she had conducted were very positive. Families told her that the vouchers factored into their weekly food budget, and that thanks to the scheme "*they were trying new fruits and vegetables*," quoting the example of one woman who said she had never tried blueberries before using the vouchers, because they are so expensive at supermarkets.

The benefits of this kind of voucher scheme are disputed. In the case of Healthy Start, some deem the interventions greatly valuable (see, e.g. Lucas, Jessiman, and Cameron 2015), whilst others contend that there has not been a significant overall increase in consumption of fruit and vegetables for target families (see Scantlebury et al. 2018), which is one of the intervention's stated core aims. It is agreed in the available literature, nonetheless, that food subsidies such as these can provide an important "nutritional safety net" (McFadden et al. 2014, 624) for vulnerable families, and as such, should not be disregarded. This being said, Healthy Start and Rose Vouchers offer another interesting example not only of how MEW plays out in the everyday lives of people, but also how different policy domains intersect with each other. Questioning the idea that behaviour change can be achieved by giving more information to 'target groups' is also useful here. Particularly for the case of nutritional knowledge, in which often too many actors assert themselves as authorities in the discourse (Kimura et al. 2014, 43; Flowers and Swan 2016, 2–3), assuming that people do not know 'what is best for them' needs to be assessed. As shown by Louise's comment above, and this brief exploration of the Rose Voucher scheme, lack of knowledge is not always a problem, but lack of access can be. Further, the stigma associated with being perceived as a 'target parent' (e.g. Wenham 2016; McArthur and Winkworth 2017), and to receive certain welfare benefits, particularly food subsidies (e.g. Garthwaite 2016), also seems to not be always addressed by those implementing the schemes.

My interview with Louise and our exchanges throughout the year I spent at Ladybird thus made me further reflect about the limitations of family intervention policies, the fact that increased knowledge does not necessarily lead to 'better choices' (e.g. see Cummins 2005; Caraher and Dowler 2007; Dowler and O'Connor 2012; Betty 2013; Ulijaszek and McLennan 2016; Evans 2017), as well as emphasising the much more pressing matters that might prevent parents from providing 'good food' for their children. Again, we can see that the universal approaches advanced in policy interventions very rarely take into account the particulars of the situations they are applied to. Louise related her financial constraints to me, but also her lived experience of using the Vouchers:

> I think, especially for me, my budget is a lot tighter now because of the nursery thing,[9] because I'm paying for it... So if I go to the market and get lots of veg and fruit [using the Rose Vouchers] that's us fed for the week, with all the fruit, some greens, small things like that, [and] then I can live like on £10 a week [...] There is one stand [in the market], that's literally the only one I go to [...] because I literally don't know where else does it [accepting the Rose Vouchers]. And the one fruit one that's at the front of the market, they used to do it but they stopped it, and now I don't know if they're doing it again. The one right at the front... and they stopped doing it, and yeah... it was a bit embarrassing, but I don't know if they're doing it now, I haven't tried it again.

Further, the challenges Louise faced at her and Emma's accommodation reveal some of the other constraints parents may face when feeding their children. Indeed, lack of access to adequate housing was one of the prevailing conversation topics among many of the parents at the children's centre. This came up in conversation with Sharon and Marie, two single mothers who also lived in temporary accommodation and used the Rose Voucher scheme:

> Sharon [Trevor's mother] and Marie [Lea and Blake's mother] talk about some of the issues they have been experiencing with housing. Since Trevor was born [a year and a half ago], he and Sharon have been living at a hostel [provided to her by the council as temporary accommodation]. Marie empathises, as she has also been in the same situation for over two years. This isn't the first time she has expressed her frustration, or spoken about

the impact that living in a small hostel room with two very active infants has had on her mental health [...] Since I know that both Sharon and Marie use Rose Vouchers, I ask them about their experience with the scheme. Both say it's been very useful to them... [more general comments] Marie interrupts the conversation to remind herself out loud that she needs to use her vouchers soon because they're about to expire. She then turns to me saying that she shouldn't waste them because her children love fruit: "Blake and Lea can eat a whole box of blueberries or strawberries in one go, but they're so expensive! One box of strawberries costs £2 at Tesco's!" she says – fieldnotes, July 2017.

Bringing the challenges these women face to the fore is a productive way of explaining why eating 'healthy food' might become a secondary concern among financially vulnerable families, but it also shows that these mothers want to be able to feed their children well (both by their own and by official standards). Based on my interactions with Louise, Sharon, Marie, and many of the other women I met at the children's centre, it is clear that most parents did not lack information or knowledge about children's (and adults') nutritional needs, but are rather faced with a number of structural constraints, whether it is inadequate housing, a limited budget to buy food, or a combination of these and other factors. It is important to note, furthermore, that a policy discourse that centres predominantly on the dissemination of nutritional messages and parental accountability is particularly harmful to women.[10]

In the Canadian context, for example, Frank (2015) shows that socioeconomically vulnerable mothers' experiences of breastfeeding were not adequately contextualised in policy and mainstream discourse. The women in her study were very aware of the benefits of exclusive breastfeeding (2015, 195–96), yet there were a number of limitations posed by their material circumstances that impacted mothers' (self) perceived or actual abilities to breastfeed their babies (ibid., 191). Frank makes a link between women's experiences of a 'compromised foodway' (e.g. restricted food budgets, issues with gaining access to food) and what they thought of the quality and amount of breastmilk they could produce, as well as how nutritious their breastmilk would be (ibid., 198). And, as others have noted, the moralisation of motherhood in relation to feeding practices is exacerbated for the case of breastfeeding (e.g. Faircloth 2013; Tomori, Palmquist, and Dowling 2016).

Similarly, O'Connell and Brannen (2016) contend that an emphasis on 'parenting styles' as determinants of children's health continues to reinforce the assumption that all "parents are willing and able to prioritise nutrition" (2016, 81–82), recreating a culture of 'parental blame,' particularly harmful to mothers. A more detailed analysis of foodwork using a gender lens will be provided in the following chapter, however, it is important to note here that the socio-economic constraints that impact child feeding practices disproportionately affect mothers – not least of all because they often sacrifice their own food intake to protect their children (Harden and Dickson 2015, 386; Child Poverty Action Group and Royal College of Paediatrics and Child Health (RCPCH) 2017, 6; O'Connell, Knight, and Brannen

2019, 107–8, 127). This again often gets left out of policy discussions. Further, it is the morally charged nature of food and parenting interventions that also leads to arbitrary results; 'target groups' are very aware of their position as subjects of interventions (e.g. Gillies 2007; Wenham 2016) and, as such, resist them. As Louise told me in our interview:

> *Lots of people judge you for being incapable of leading your own life. But I think, for me [...] from a young age I was already cooking for myself, because I cooked for my family...from like the age of nine, I used to cook for everyone [...] I've always known how to cook, and I've always known how to fend for myself. And I don't know, it's probably a mind-set thing. I think people look at me and probably think I don't know how to cook.*

Louise's account powerfully demonstrates the limitations of the paternalistic assumption that 'target groups' are not aware that they are being intervened upon through policy and by official actors. This awareness, in turn, discourages engagement with interventions, leading on the one hand to further patchiness in policy results, but also to the marginalisation of those that might need and benefit from accessing some level of support from available services, even if these provisions are not perfect (see, e.g. McArthur and Winkworth 2017).

Health, Nutrition and Exercise for the Really Young (HENRY)

The tensions that arise when food and parenting are viewed as moral categories were also evident during my participation in a session of the 'HENRY Approach' (introduced in Chapter 1), which I observed and took part in at a different children's centre in the borough. HENRY was developed in 2007, promoted in England and Wales through local public health departments, NHS Trusts, and early years services (Roberts 2015, 88). The programme has been rolled out "as part of universal services in children's centres in disadvantaged areas in 36 Local Authorities" (ibid.), recognising the link between obesity and socio-economic inequality in its mission statement, as well as the need to make the program 'culturally sensitive,' so as to be able to engage with families from diverse backgrounds, and who might experience barriers in accessing preventative health care services (ibid., 91). In line with these aims, the group that attended the session I took part in reflected the objective of engaging with this demographic. None of the six participants were British (one was Polish, another Romanian, two were Slovakian, and two Brazilian), all were stay-at-home mothers of working-class background, and all were married, except for one of the Brazilian women, who was a single parent. The session was run by Anne and Nadia – Nadia knew Robert, the extended services manager at Ladybird, who introduced us.

Nadia was not there yet when I arrived to the session I was invited to partake in. My first encounter of the day was with Anne, who introduced herself as the community development manager at the children's centre. While we waited for Nadia to arrive, Anne also told me a bit about her career path, saying she started as an early years practitioner and then decided to switch to community development when she *"realised the complexity of families' needs"* in the borough. Nadia arrived shortly after. In preparation for the parents' arrival, I helped her hang some of the course materials, and organise the families' course packs on a table.

After the participants arrived and took their seats, Nadia announced the themes that the group would work on that day: portion sizes and reading food packaging. Following the holistic model advocated in the 'HENRY Approach,' Nadia explained that it is important to keep in mind that eating healthy is not only about the "physical aspect" but also about our mental and/or emotional states.

And indeed, although Anne and Nadia structured the discussion around the topic of 'healthy eating,' some of the women seemed to prefer (or need) to talk about the emotional struggles of parenting, as well as some of the family dynamics that the HENRY model encouraged them to think about as conducive or unfavourable to achieving a 'healthy lifestyle.' In my fieldnotes I noted:

> *Elvira [the Polish woman] spends about 20 minutes sharing some deep concerns she has about her two-year-old daughter's behaviour. She explains that the girl has recently been throwing serious tantrums, and that the previous night during dinner she screamed and cried for almost two hours (making Elvira concerned that the neighbours would complain and "call the police"). She says she feels extremely anxious about her child's behaviour, particularly when she's in public, saying she feels very ashamed when people stare at them. She's also very worried that, because of these extreme tantrums, her daughter might be denied a place at nursery. We all listen attentively, and Anne responds to her concerns in an understanding manner, telling her she should not care what people think and that the best thing to do is to talk to the child and ask her what she's feeling. Elvira says that that's what she tries, but that when her daughter is "screaming at the top of her lungs it's difficult" [...] Anne eventually steers the conversation back to the topics of the session, telling Elvira that if she needs to talk about this further they should discuss it at the end of the session, or any other time she wants – fieldnotes, March 2017.*

Elvira's distressed account echoes some of the tensions and anxieties that emerge at the intersection of food and mothering as moral categories. Elvira's worry that her daughter's cries could lead to a police intervention also speaks of the added scrutiny that working-class and ethnic minority parents are often faced with. Elvira's experience mirrors what other scholars have also pointed out: that working-class parents are at much higher risk of being judged and even criminalised in day-to-day occurrences (e.g. Gillies 2007), and that many migrant families face deep tensions around integration and belonging in the neighbourhoods they live in (e.g. Wessendorf 2014).

As Lee (2011) contends, an overlap between policy domains (public health and family intervention) has fuelled moral claims about different parenting and, in the case of this book, feeding practices, to the extent that "social problems have become medicalized [and] understood as best addressed via…scientific/medical insights and associated inventions directed at individuals" (2011, 3). Biomedical paradigms of health and eating can erase the social and caring dimension of feeding practices – the universalism of public health overshadows the particularism of feeding and caring through food. Food does not only fulfil nutritional and functional purposes in the everyday lives of families, it is also a channel through which social relations (and power dynamics between adults and children) are developed and negotiated.

Given the emphasis these approaches have on 'improving parenting styles' and on shaping children's habits for the future, the question remains whether these policy domains take children's present experiences into account – is children's food policy for children, or for 'better parenting'?

Notes

1 On the other side of the coin, these entrenched assumptions might lead to parents who *do* need support, guidance, or to be part of a community, to be left out if they are (or are perceived as) privileged. As will be shown in Chapter 6 of this book, most parents, especially mothers, share similar concerns about their children's eating regardless of their socio-economic or ethnic background, or their levels of knowledge and skills on food and eating. This points to a further mismatch between policy aims and people's needs.
2 There was an underlying assumption from Ladybird staff that the free meal provided at the end of each class acted as an important incentive for some of the parents to participate.
3 Sharp knives were used sometimes, but these were restricted to the kitchen area for child safety reasons.
4 These were often game-card style didactic materials; for example, flashcards of certain food items were given to parents with ingredient lists in the back, with which they were taught what to look out for when reading food packaging.
5 For instance, by making their own plant-based version of the 'Eatwell Plate' (now 'Eatwell Guide') designed by the NHS (Figure 1.1 in Chapter 1).
6 British supermarket chain known for its low-cost frozen foods selection.
7 An emphasis on helping single, young mothers through targeted interventions is pervasive in this policy rhetoric (see, e.g. Gillies 2007).
8 "Healthy Start [HS] provides vouchers which can be exchanged for infant formula, liquid cow's milk, fresh or frozen fruit and vegetables, and free vitamins to families that include a pregnant woman or children under the age of four years. Families in receipt of Income Support, income-based Jobseeker's Allowance, income-related Employment and Support Allowance, pregnant women aged under eighteen and families receiving Child Tax Credit and with an income of £16,190 or less are eligible for HS" (Lucas, Jessiman, and Cameron 2015, 458).
9 Louise had started her bakery apprenticeship at this time and had to pay for Emma's childcare on the days on which she was working.
10 This will be explored at length in Chapter 6.

References

Albon, Deborah. 2005. 'Approaches to the Study of Children, Food and Sweet Eating: A Review of the Literature'. *Early Child Development and Care* 175 (5): 407–17. https:// doi.org/10.1080/0300443042000244055.

Alexandra Rose Charity. 2018a. 'How Rose Vouchers Work'. Alexandra Rose Charity. 2018. https://www.alexandrarose.org.uk/how-rose-vouchers-work.

———. 2018b. 'Our History'. Alexandra Rose Charity. 2018. https://www.alexandrarose. org.uk/our-history.

Ashton, John R., John Middleton, and Tim Lang. 2014. 'Open Letter to Prime Minister David Cameron on Food Poverty in the UK'. *The Lancet* 383 (9929): 1631. https://doi. org/10.1016/S0140-6736(14)60536-5.

Bacchi, Carol. 2010. 'Poststructuralism, Discourse and Problematization: Implications for Gender Mainstreaming'. *KVINDER, KØN & FORSKNING* 4: 62–72.

Bacchi, Carol, and Susan Goodwin. 2016. *Poststructural Policy Analysis: A Guide to Practice*. New York: Palgrave Macmillan.

Baez, Benjamin, and Susan Talburt. 2008. 'Governing for Responsibility and with Love: Parents and Children between Home and School'. *Educational Theory* 58 (1): 25–43.

Betty, A. L. 2013. 'Using Financial Incentives to Increase Fruit and Vegetable Consumption in the UK: Increasing Fruit and Vegetable Consumption'. *Nutrition Bulletin* 38 (4): 414–20. https://doi.org/10.1111/nbu.12062.

Brannen, Julia, and Rebecca O'Connell. 2022. 'Thinking about the Future: Young People in Low-Income Families'. *Societies* 12 (3): 86. https://doi.org/10.3390/soc12030086.

Caraher, Martin, and Elizabeth Dowler. 2007. 'Food Projects in London: Lessons for Policy and Practice—A Hidden Sector and the Need for "More Unhealthy Puddings… Sometimes"'. *Health Education Journal* 66 (2): 188–205.

Child Poverty Action Group and Royal College of Paediatrics and Child Health (RCPCH). 2017. 'Poverty and Child Health: Views from the Frontline'. London: Child Poverty Action Group. http://www.cpag.org.uk/sites/default/files/pdf%20RCPCH.pdf.

Chilton, Mariana, and Donald Rose. 2009. 'A Rights-Based Approach to Food Insecurity in the United States'. *American Journal of Public Health* 99 (7): 1203–11. https://doi. org/10.2105/AJPH.2007.130229.

Costa, Sandrine, Lydia Zepeda, and Lucie Sirieix. 2014. 'Exploring the Social Value of Organic Food: A Qualitative Study in France: Exploring the Social Value of Organic Food'. *International Journal of Consumer Studies* 38 (3): 228–37. https://doi.org/10.1111/ ijcs.12100.

Cummins, S. 2005. 'Large Scale Food Retailing as an Intervention for Diet and Health: Quasi-Experimental Evaluation of a Natural Experiment'. *Journal of Epidemiology & Community Health* 59 (12): 1035–40. https://doi.org/10.1136/jech.2004.029843.

Dowler, Elizabeth. 2002. 'Food and Poverty in Britain: Rights and Responsibilities'. *Social Policy & Administration* 36 (6): 698–717.

Dowler, Elizabeth A., and Deirdre O'Connor. 2012. 'Rights-Based Approaches to Addressing Food Poverty and Food Insecurity in Ireland and UK'. *Social Science & Medicine* 74 (1): 44–51. https://doi.org/10.1016/j.socscimed.2011.08.036.

Eisenberg, Merrill. 2011. 'Medical Anthropology and Public Policy'. In *A Companion to Medical Anthropology*, edited by Merrill Singer and Pamela I. Erickson, 93–116. London: Blackwell Publishing Ltd.

Evans, Charlotte Elizabeth Louise. 2017. 'Sugars and Health: A Review of Current Evidence and Future Policy'. *Proceedings of the Nutrition Society* 76 (03): 400–7. https://doi. org/10.1017/S0029665116002846.

Faircloth, Charlotte. 2013. '"What Feels Right": Affect, Emotion, and the Limitations of Infant-Feeding Policy'. *Journal of Women, Politics & Policy* 34 (4): 345–58. https://doi. org/10.1080/1554477X.2013.835678.

Flowers, Rick, and Elaine Swan, eds. 2016. *Food Pedagogies*. London: Routledge.

Food Ethics Council. 2017. 'The Beginning of the End of Cheap Food? How Should We Prepare for Food Inflation and True Cost Food?' London: Food Ethics Council. http://www.foodethicscouncil.org/uploads/publications/170131%20The%20beginning%20of%20the%20end%20of%20cheap%20food_FINAL.pdf.

Foucault, Michel. 1978. *The History of Sexuality, Vol. 1: An Introduction.* New York: Pantheon Books.

———. 1991. 'Governmentality'. In *The Foucault Effect: Studies in Governmentality, with Two Lectures by and an Interview with Michel Foucault*, edited by Graham Burchell, Colin Gordon, and Peter Miller. Chicago: University of Chicago Press.

Frank, Lesley. 2015. 'Exploring Infant Feeding Pratices In Food Insecure Households: What Is The Real Issue?' *Food and Foodways* 23 (3): 186–209. https://doi.org/10.1080/07409 710.2015.1066223.

Garthwaite, Kayleigh. 2016. *Hunger Pains. Life inside Foodbank Britain.* Bristol: Policy Press.

Gillies, Val. 2007. *Marginalised Mothers: Exploring Working-Class Experiences of Parenting.* London: Routlegde.

Goodwin, Sabine. 2022. 'Food Aid Charities Fear the Worst as the Cost of Living Crisis Takes Hold'. *BMJ*, February, o416. https://doi.org/10.1136/bmj.o416.

Gupta, Akhil. 2012. *Red Tape Bureaucracy, Structural Violence, and Poverty in India.* Durham: Duke University Press.

Guthman, Julie. 2011. '"If They Only Knew": The Unbearable Whiteness of Alternative Food'. In *Cultivating Food Justice*, edited by Alison Hope Alkon and Julian Agyeman, 263–282. Cambridge: The MIT Press.

Harden, Jeni, and Adele Dickson. 2015. 'Low-Income Mothers' Food Practices with Young Children: A Qualitative Longitudinal Study'. *Health Education Journal* 74 (4): 381–91. https://doi.org/10.1177/0017896914535378.

Harman, Vicki, Charlotte Faircloth, and Benedetta Cappellini. 2019. 'Introduction'. In *Feeding Children Inside and Outside the Home: Critical Perspectives*, edited by Vicki Harman, Benedetta Cappellini, and Charlotte Faircloth, 1–8. Abingdon: Routledge.

Harper, Breeze A. 2011. 'Vegans of Color, Racialized Embodiment, and Problematics of the "Exotic"'. In *Cultivating Food Justice*, edited by Alison Hope Alkon and Julian Agyeman, 221–238. Cambridge: The MIT Press.

Jones, Nicholas R. V., Annalijn I. Conklin, Marc Suhrcke, and Pablo Monsivais. 2014. 'The Growing Price Gap between More and Less Healthy Foods: Analysis of a Novel Longitudinal UK Dataset'. Edited by Harry Zhang. *PLoS ONE* 9 (10): 1–7. https://doi.org/10.1371/journal.pone.0109343.

Kimura, Aya H., Charlotte Biltekoff, Jessica Mudry, and Jessica Hayes-Conroy. 2014. 'Nutrition as a Project'. *Gastronomica: The Journal of Critical Food Studies* 14 (3): 34–55.

Lang, Tim. 2019. 'No-Deal Food Planning in UK Brexit'. *The Lancet*, August. https://doi.org/10.1016/S0140-6736(19)31769-6.

Lang, Tim, and Geof Rayner. 2010. 'Corporate Responsibility in Public Health: The Government's Invitation to the Food Industry to Fund Social Marketing on Obesity Is Risky'. *BMJ: British Medical Journal* 341 (7764): 110–11.

Lee, Ellie. 2011. 'Medicalization and Moral Claims: Health Care Policies Concerning the Family and Their Effects on the Moral Understanding of the Family'. Symposium: 'Between relational autonomy and trust', Goettingen University, Germany, July. https://blogs.kent.ac.uk/parentingculturestudies/files/2013/11/EI-pages-paper-1-Gottingen-Lee.pdf.Lee, Ellie, Jennie Bristow, Charlotte Faircloth, and Jan Macvarish. 2014. *Parenting Culture Studies*. Basingstoke: Palgrave Macmillan.

Lucas, Patricia J., Tricia Jessiman, and Ailsa Cameron. 2015. 'Healthy Start: The Use of Welfare Food Vouchers by Low-Income Parents in England'. *Social Policy and Society* 14 (03): 457–69. https://doi.org/10.1017/S1474746415000020.

Lupton, Deborah. 1995. *The Imperative of Health: Public Health and the Regulated Body*. London: SAGE Publications.

Maher, JaneMaree, Suzanne Fraser, and Jo Lindsay. 2010. 'Between Provisioning and Consuming?: Children, Mothers and "Childhood Obesity"'. *Health Sociology Review* 19 (3): 304–16.

Maher, JaneMaree, Suzanne Fraser, and Jan Wright. 2010. 'Framing the Mother: Childhood Obesity, Maternal Responsibility and Care'. *Journal of Gender Studies* 19 (3): 233–47. https://doi.org/10.1080/09589231003696037.

McArthur, Morag, and Gail Winkworth. 2017. 'Give Them a Break: How Stigma Impacts on Younger Mothers Accessing Early and Supportive Help in Australia'. *The British Journal of Social Work* 0 (August): 1–19. https://doi.org/10.1093/bjsw/bcx075.

McFadden, Alison, Josephine M. Green, Victoria Williams, Jenny McLeish, Felicia McCormick, Julia Fox-Rushby, and Mary J Renfrew. 2014. 'Can Food Vouchers Improve Nutrition and Reduce Health Inequalities in Low-Income Mothers and Young Children: A Multi-Method Evaluation of the Experiences of Beneficiaries and Practitioners of the Healthy Start Programme in England'. *BMC Public Health* 14 (1). https://doi.org/10.1186/1471-2458-14-148.

Morris, Kate, and Brid Featherstone. 2010. 'Investing in Children, Regulating Parents, Thinking Family: A Decade of Tensions and Contradictions'. *Social Policy and Society* 9 (04): 557–66. https://doi.org/10.1017/S1474746410000278.

Moss, Peter, and Pat Petrie. 2000. *From Children's Services to Children's Spaces*. London: Routledge/Falmer.

Mosse, David. 2005. *Cultivating Development: An Ethnography of Aid Policy and Practice*. London: Pluto Press.

O'Connell, Rebecca and Julia Brannen. 2016. *Food, Families and Work*. London: Bloomsbury.

O'Connell, Rebecca, Abigail Knight, and Julia Brannen. 2019. *Living Hand to Mouth: Children and Food in Low-Income Families*. London: Child Poverty Action Group.

O'Connell, Rebecca, Charlie Owen, Matt Padley, Antonia Simon, and Julia Brannen. 2018. 'Which Types of Family Are at Risk of Food Poverty in the UK? A Relative Deprivation Approach'. *Social Policy and Society*, February, 1–18. https://doi.org/10.1017/S1474746418000015.

Powell, Martin. 2014. *Understanding the Mixed Economy of Welfare*. Bristol: The Policy Press.

Power, Michael. 1999. *The Audit Society: Rituals of Verification*. Oxford: Oxford University Press.

Procacci, Giovanna. 1991. 'Social Economy and the Government of Poverty'. In *The Foucault Effect: Studies in Governmentality, with Two Lectures by and an Interview with Michel Foucault*, edited by Graham Burchell, Colin Gordon, and Peter Miller. Chicago: University of Chicago Press 151–169.

Randall, Vicky. 2000. *The Politics of Child Daycare in Britain*. Oxford: Oxford University Press.

Roberts, Kim. 2015. 'Growing Up Not out: The HENRY Approach to Preventing Childhood Obesity'. *British Journal of Obesity* 1 (3): 87–92.

Rose, Nikolas. 1996. 'Governing "Advanced" Liberal Democracies'. In *Foucault and Political Reason. Liberalism, Neo-Liberalism and Rationalities of Government*, edited by Andrew Barry, Thomas Osborne, and Nikolas Rose. London: Routledge 37–64.

————. 1999. *Powers of Freedom: Reframing Political Thought*. Cambridge: Cambridge University Press.

Scantlebury, Rachel Jane, Alison Moody, Oyinlola Oyebode, and Jennifer Susan Mindell. 2018. 'Has the UK Healthy Start Voucher Scheme Been Associated with an Increased Fruit and Vegetable Intake among Target Families? Analysis of Health Survey for England Data, 2001–2014'. *Journal of Epidemiology and Community Health* 72 (7): 623–29. https://doi.org/10.1136/jech-2017-209954.

Semple, Tara. 2022. *Hipsterism: A Paradigm of Modernity*. Wiesbaden: Springer VS.

Shore, Cris. 2017. 'Audit Culture and the Politics of Responsibility: Beyond Neoliberal Responsibilization?' In *Competing Responsibilities: The Ethics and Politics of Contemporary Life*, edited by Susanna Trnka and Catherine Trundle, 96–117. Durham: Duke University Press.

Stewart, John, and Kieron Walsh. 1992. 'Change in the Management of Public Services'. *Public Administration* 70 (4): 499–518.

Tomori, Cecilia, Aunchalee E. L. Palmquist, and Sally Dowling. 2016. 'Contested Moral Landscapes: Negotiating Breastfeeding Stigma in Breastmilk Sharing, Nighttime Breastfeeding, and Long-Term Breastfeeding in the U.S. and the U.K.' *Social Science & Medicine* 168 (November): 178–85. https://doi.org/10.1016/j.socscimed.2016.09.014.

Ulijaszek, Stanley J., and Amy K. McLennan. 2016. 'Framing Obesity in UK Policy from the Blair Years, 1997-2015: The Persistence of Individualistic Approaches despite Overwhelming Evidence of Societal and Economic Factors, and the Need for Collective Responsibility'. *Obesity Reviews* 17 (5): 397–411. https://doi.org/10.1111/obr.12386.

Wake, Melissa. 2018. 'The Failure of Anti-Obesity Programmes in Schools'. *BMJ* 360 (February): 1–2. https://doi.org/10.1136/bmj.k507.

Wenham, Aniela. 2016. '"I Know I'm a Good Mum – No One Can Tell Me Different." Young Mothers Negotiating a Stigmatised Identity through Time'. *Families, Relationships and Societies* 5 (1): 127–44. https://doi.org/10.1332/204674315X14193466354732.

Wessendorf, Susanne. 2014. '"Being Open, but Sometimes Closed". Conviviality in a Super-Diverse London Neighbourhood'. *European Journal of Cultural Studies* 17 (4): 392–405.

6   Mothers and foodwork

This chapter will centre on an analysis of mothers' foodwork, understood as a broad range of activities, including planning menus, purchasing food, cooking, cleaning after meals, and assuming responsibility for one's family's diet (Allen and Sachs 2012, 1; O'Connell and Brannen 2016, 11). For this discussion, I will draw predominantly from semi-structured interviews carried out in participants' homes. The way in which foodwork can be understood as part of an 'intensive mothering' (Faircloth 2014) culture will also be examined.

To explore how the themes of responsibility and control overlapped in discussion with mothers, I will return to Foucault's idea of governmentality as "diffuse" (Foucault 1991; Lupton 1995, 9), meaning that it is exerted from the top-down, but also between individuals who surveil each other and surveil themselves. By focusing on the theme of responsibility on a micro-level, I aim to show the contrast between the universalism of food and family intervention policies examined in Chapter 1 and the particularism of feeding children and caring through food.

Finally, and drawing again from the work of Mikhail Bakhtin (1986) presented in Chapter 4, the way in which children and mothers relate to each other through food and eating practices will be discussed. By emphasising the circularity of language and practices described by Bakhtin's notion of the dialogic (1986), I will show that it is not only children that respond to and reinterpret their parents' views on food and eating, it is also the adults that react to (and sometimes adopt) their children's newly acquired preferences and knowledge. Importantly, this highlights the centrality of not only language, but also practice in Bakhtin's dialogic (Albon and Rosen 2014, 9; Marjanovic-Shane and White 2014, 120); children reinterpret norms and behaviours from their homes and school, bringing them into each context. This has important implications for how we think of children's agency, and their role in influencing the social worlds they inhabit, rather than being passive learners.

Feeding children: women's work?

> *M-U-M, M-U-M, mum is my best friend! She helps me cook, and read a book, and the fun just never ends! – nursery rhyme sang at Ladybird Nursery and Children's Centre on Mother's Day, 2017.*

DOI: 10.4324/9781003297642-7

During the year that I conducted fieldwork, feeding children was predominantly women's work. Within Ladybird, all staff members who were directly involved in feeding children during mealtimes were female, except for one male nursery teacher. The council-funded courses and interventions discussed in the previous chapter were exclusively attended by women, although some fathers attended the 'stay-and-play' sessions at the children's centre. Throughout this book, I have also discussed how class is implicated in the construction of food and parenting as moral categories. Yet, gender is another important category to bring into this discussion. Because women are still largely responsible for feeding children, I argue that it is mothers' (rather than fathers') practices which are more often subjected to the scrutiny of official actors, as also noted by O'Connell and Brannen (2016, 82) and others (Harman, Faircloth, and Cappellini 2019; S. Elliott and Bowen 2018; Maher, JaneMaree, Fraser, Suzanne, and Lindsay 2010; Maher, Fraser, and Wright 2010. For an exploration of parents' feeding anxieties in the Polish context, see Boni 2023).

Although I had not expected foodwork to be shared completely equally between men and women when I first started my research, I did find it surprising that this is still such a predominantly female domain, particularly in a city as cosmopolitan and diverse as London. This did not only seem to be the case within families, but also at a professional level. Within the borough, the actors I encountered who promoted children's food or healthy eating initiatives were also all women. When staff members at Ladybird spoke about parents' feeding practices, it was assumed that mothers were generally in charge of this, suggesting that a strong link still exists between food, care, and 'hegemonic femininity' (Cairns and Johnston 2015) – as also indicated by the lyrics of the nursery rhyme above.

Assuming that women are instinctively caring, and know how and what to feed children, has problematic implications for both women and men. If a mother's practices were being commented on or intervened upon, it seemed that the implicit assumption underlying this need for intervention was to fill a gap that should not exist: all women should know what and how to cook. Women have to opt out of cooking, whereas men can opt in. In the case of fathers, the assumption was that men are much more at a loss and needed to be instructed not only on what and how to feed their children, but also on how to care. I observed how these assumptions shaped the interactions between Ladybird staff and the three fathers that regularly attended the children's centre. Nonetheless, the same assumptions seemed prevalent also in the accounts of the women I interviewed. Whilst the conspicuous absence of male voices in this thesis is also indicative of what I have argued thus far – that feeding infants and children remains a predominantly female domain – examining how official and mainstream discourses and practices operate to exclude men from this sphere is important. Although exploring this topic at length is beyond the scope of this chapter, I hope it will become evident that foodwork, in many instances, continues to reproduce traditional ideas and norms both about femininity *and* masculinity, which can negatively impact women and men alike.

Being in control (i): the 'right' environment, menu plans, and juggling time

This section focuses on women's discussions about controlling their children's diets, not only in terms of nutrition but also in terms of other practical elements related to feeding children, such as having a 'right' eating environment, planning meals, purchasing food, as well as conceding to some of their children's desires. The topic of mothers' control and surveillance of children's eating habits has been at the centre of scholarly attention, both how adults and children negotiate these power dynamics (e.g. O'Connell and Brannen 2014; Boni 2019) as well as how power is not only enacted by parents on children, but more broadly by the state and other institutions on parents (e.g. Allison 1991; Afflerback et al. 2013; Faircloth and Murray 2015). I will predominantly focus on the accounts of three women: Rose, Vivian, and Adriana. Allen and Sachs contend that, "Women are occupied in and preoccupied with food on a daily basis, irrespective of class, culture, or ethnicity" (2007, 2). Whilst in the previous chapter I examined how women's inter-actions with official discourses and practices can vary significantly depending on their class or ethnic backgrounds, in this chapter I will emphasise that gender (as the commonality between these participants) plays a decisive role in shaping their experiences of foodwork.

Rose is a white, English woman, who was a stay-at-home mother at the time of our interview. Her husband ran an events production company, and they lived in a mortgaged flat in a new-built complex in the borough, with their two children Susie (four-years-old, whom I got to know at Ladybird) and Toby (two-and-half-years-old).

Vivian is of mixed European and East Asian background and was brought up in England. Although at the time of our interview she was on maternity leave after the birth of her second child, when we first met at Ladybird she worked full time at a film production company. Her partner, a European migrant, worked freelance. They lived in a flat that they owned in a council estate tower-block, also in the borough, with their son Fred (three-years-old) and their new-born son.

Finally, Adriana is a first-generation migrant from South America; she and her husband had been living in London for ten years at the time of our interview. She had trained as a nurse in her country of origin and had previously worked as a childminder since her arrival to the U.K., although at the time of our interview she was not employed. Her husband, who had studied law in his birth country, now worked as supervisor at a cleaning company. They live in a council flat in the borough (we did not discuss whether the family owned or rented the flat) with their eldest son (twenty-one-years-old) and their daughter Maria (four-years-old).

In the conversations I will present here, the themes of responsibility and sur-veillance are prevalent. These themes came up naturally; I had planned to ask participants' views about whose responsibility it is to provide 'healthy food' to chil-dren (whatever healthy food might have meant to them), and to teach them about it, yet their accounts often led to discussions about how *they* felt particularly responsi-ble for their children's diets. Their narratives also emphasise that feeding children is not simply a matter of providing adequate nutrition, but encompasses a wide range of other aims that are not only practical, but also tied to a number of moral dimensions. As Harman, Faircloth, and Cappellini contend, the moralisation of eating and mothering are deeply interlinked (2019, 4). They suggest that notions of 'good food' and 'good mothering' are usually tied together, and surveillance of children's eating habits is often also related to women's self-surveillance (ibid., 1). I thus conceptualise foodwork as a particular way of 'doing gender' (DeVault 1991, 118; Cairns and Johnston 2015, 25) and 'doing family' (Brannen, O'Connell, and Mooney 2013, 428) that reproduces what Cairns and Johnston have termed 'hegemonic femininity':

> The defining feature of hegemonic femininity is its relation to an unequal gender order where power is unequally distributed [...] the performance of hegemonic food femininities can engender social and emotional rewards for women – as seen in positive evaluations of the 'good mother' who carefully monitors and regulates her child's diet. At the same time, femininities become hegemonic precisely because they serve to uphold patriarchal relations of power – such as the expectation that women are 'naturally' caring and thus primarily responsible for the labour of social reproduction, prioritizing the needs of others before their own needs.
>
> (2015, 27–28)

Although hegemonic femininity is entrenched in many Euro-American contexts, it does not remain unchallenged. As will become apparent through participants' own accounts, the constant negotiation of roles and expectations about feeding children can contest some of the structural inequalities described by Cairns and Johnston. At the same time, hegemonic femininity is still strongly reproduced in households and in public life, and through myriad practices, particularly when linked to a desire to fulfil normative ideals of what constitutes a family meal.

Parental control of children's eating habits in recent decades has also been tied to the expansion of an 'intensive mothering' (Hays 1996) or 'intensive parenting' (Lee et al. 2014) culture, understood as a 'style' of parenting informed by a mainstream belief that there is currently enough expertise and information about childrearing available to parents, so parents can be considered fully responsible for their children's life outcomes (Faircloth 2014, 31). Many of the ideas, worries, and aspirations that participants shared with me with regards to their feeding practices mirror this preoccupation to be in control of, and intervene in, their children's lives, looking towards 'expert knowledge' for guidance (Faircloth 2014).

Like most, if not all, parents that I spoke with during the year that I conducted fieldwork, Vivian, Rose, and Adriana made their desire (and concern with) feeding their children 'healthy food' quite explicit. Alongside this goal, they expressed a strong sense of duty and an awareness that their own habits had an impact on their children. Vivian, for example, explained in our interview that she worried that Fred might not develop a varied diet: "*I'd be heartbroken if he turned into a kid that only ate fish fingers and chips,*" she jokingly said, "*it may happen, but it really will break my heart!*" I asked her if she was worried about any 'external influences' that Fred might encounter as he grew up, something that she had voiced during a focused group discussion conducted with other mothers at Ladybird:

FV: *You mentioned [in the focused group discussion] being a bit worried about the 'external influences' that he gets...*
VIVIAN: *Yeah, and my own, you know, I think I grew up with some bad habits... I look back on it now and I think, ok yeah... you know, we all have bad habits when it comes to food, and I am worried about passing them on. I'm not that great with vegetables myself, eating them regularly, and eating them fresh, so I'm conscious of that as well [...] What matters to me is that he eats a mixed diet, healthy, that he understands...you know, healthy foods, it doesn't always have to be healthy, there can be treats, there are sweet things, but to get him into good habits, with healthy food and a mixed diet.*

Rose expressed a similar view about her role in teaching Susie and Toby about healthy eating, also reflecting on her own mother's practices:

ROSE: *My mum was always eating healthily and she was always cooking from scratch, so that's what felt normal to me and that definitely impacted on my eating habits, as I've become an adult, and it just carries on doesn't it? So I think that's important, that kind of role modelling of thinking about food, being healthy, all these kinds of things.*
FV: *So do you feel responsible for this?*
ROSE: *Oh yes, definitely, definitely. I think it's a dual thing, it's about the health of their bodies now, and providing the right balance, but also, and possibly more importantly, the behavioural aspect...essentially for the rest of their lives, I think if you've grown up with it kind of being a normal thing, eating lots of fruits and vegetables, and to eat lots of whole grains and things like that...then that's what you do, and it's what you'll probably like, whereas if you've grown up eating lots of crap, essentially, then that is what you will like as an adult so...yeah, I do feel responsibility.*

In these conversations, participants conveyed an urgency to shape the eating practices of their children in the present to guarantee their future well-being. I have already emphasised that discourses about children's food and eating are often future-oriented. In official contexts, this links to a focus on school readiness and future health outcomes (e.g. Albon 2015), a vision that was also shared by staff members at Ladybird. For the mothers I spoke with, this seemed to relate to the commonly held assumption that parenting practices are generally considered to have a lasting and definitive impact on children's futures (Harman, Faircloth, and Cappellini 2019, 6). Thus, similarly to Rose, Adriana told me:

If we love our family we need to be conscious [of their health]... that's why one brings children to this world, why one makes a family, you need to love them, take care of them, feed them healthy things so they can grow up healthy. So that they won't be a burden on society, so that they will grow up to be good men and women who will contribute to society [...] Because if they have a healthy body then they will also have a healthy mind.[1]

An awareness or (self-)consciousness with regards to one's own eating behaviour, and how these might impact on children's diets, was also echoed by Vivian, who shared her concern that she might "pass on" her "bad habits" to Fred. This has important implications with which to think about food, parenting, and governmentality.

Foucault identifies four "specific techniques that human beings use to understand themselves" (1988, 18): technologies of production, technologies of sign systems, technologies of power, and technologies of the self. The interaction between technologies of power and of the self in particular, he argues, is what constitutes governmentality (ibid., 19). Foucault's definition of technologies of the self as "types of self-examination" (1988, 46), and Foucault's and Lupton's framing of governmentality as "diffuse" (Foucault 1991; Lupton 1995), highlights that the self-surveillance that governmentality relies on to exist is intrinsic to the notion that autonomous, rational, and responsible individuals have the ability to make 'good choices' about the food they eat and feed to their children. Following this definition of governmentality as "diffuse," mothers' accounts shed light on how the surveillance of child feeding practices happens beyond institutional contexts.

The theme of responsibility was deeply tied to women's self-surveillance, revealing different moral understandings of the self and their children's future personhood. Like Rose and Vivian, Adriana expressed feeling a strong sense of responsibility for her children's eating practices:

I do think that parents are totally responsible for teaching children to eat healthy food. And [as parents] we are responsible for taking care of ourselves too [...] I try to always eat healthily and [in doing so] to also take care of them [my family].[2]

In these accounts (and similarly to what staff members described in Chapter 3), feeding children healthy food was associated with aims that are a lot less immediately tangible than providing regular nourishment. For Adriana, promoting 'healthy eating' fit into a much broader set of aspirations for her children, which linked to her hopes for them to become "*good men and women who will contribute to society.*" Being a devout Christian, this desire also seemed to be rooted in her religious ethic, which – as she explained it to me – involves the continuous improvement of the self, both to be good to others but also to ultimately honour Jesus Christ in every aspect of one's life. Indeed, Adriana brought up the topic of religion several times during our interviews, often linking it to most of her daily practices, as well as to the values that she tried to encourage within her family.

For Adriana, the physical health of her family seemed to be as important as their spiritual health. She voiced particular concern for her eldest son's weight, telling me that he was easily "tempted" by 'junk food,' but she was also worried about her husband's health, as he lived with type 2 diabetes.

Whilst the pursuit of Christian values cannot be paralleled to the kind of self-improvement and self-regulation (Mitchell 2014, 12) that prevails in most advanced liberal democracies (and indeed this comparison is beyond the scope of this chapter), it is worth exploring how notions of 'good food' overlap with other moral categories in the narratives of all the mothers I spoke with. Just as 'good food' meant good future (Christian) personhood for Adriana, 'good food' meant good future health for Rose. For Vivian, it also meant developing an appreciation for food and eating or, as she put it, "*an understanding about food.*" She said:

> *I also try and explain to him [Fred] why I'm doing it [encouraging him to eat a healthy/varied diet], because I think it's important that he learns things like, savoury comes before sweet, you know, if you eat something sweet you'll ruin your appetite, or I'm insisting on this because it's important for you to have a mixed diet.*

These considerations echo Lupton's argument that food practices (both what is eaten and how) is deeply tied to western ideals of the 'civilised body' (1996, 31), as has been discussed throughout this book. Simultaneously, regulating children's diets ties to the notion that infant bodies need to be 'civilised' and 'contained' (Lupton 2012, 39).

In Rose's, Vivian's, and Adriana's accounts the link between 'healthy eating' and normative ideas about family meals was also evident, particularly the material and social conditions necessary to achieve these standards. Vivian, for example, was apprehensive about Fred's 'eating environment.' During the home interview, she explained:

> *I suppose the other thing about food that we haven't really achieved is the environment, like this is...[gesturing to the room around us] our flat, we're still doing it up, it's a source of...quite a lot of frustration. And you know, years ago, we gutted it and we've done it up, but there's still loads of stuff that isn't sorted. And so, the living room, we've barely got any furniture and there's lots of distractions for Fred. So this table, we've only got this one table, and my partner is a freelancer so he works from home, so it's where his computer is, it's where there are toys, it's where the printer is [...] and I have this ambition in which we will have a table where, yeah, sometimes there might be a laptop, but when it's dinner time it will be stored away, and we can just sit down and have food with nothing else on the table. So we'll see...we'll see when that happens. But I really want to move all this [points at the computer/work station] because my partner, we'll be having dinner and he'll be looking at the internet, and Fred stares in...and it's something, we disagree about it, I think...I don't sit there with my laptop during dinner. I sit*

where you're sitting [head of the table] and I sit with Fred and talk, and my partner doesn't do that. Sometimes he does, sometimes he doesn't...I'm quite particular about it.

It seemed that this frustration was also rooted in what Vivian had read about the effect of children having 'screen time' during meals, something that she had also voiced during the focused group discussion. In our interview, she told me:

I did some Googling about it [screen time], and I found that when you're watching something while you're eating you're not chewing properly so they [the children] are not registering what they eat, and they don't learn to understand when their body is full and stuff like that so, I'm quite particular about...when TV happens.

I had already encountered notions about the importance of the environment in which children eat, particularly in relation to overcoming 'fussy eating,' in official discourse. Early on in my fieldwork, Joyce (the lead early years practitioner at Ladybird) and I attended a course for practitioners working in children's centres, on how to give parents advice about fussy eating and constipation. One of the recommendations that the dietician leading the class proposed was a list of "*appropriate conditions for eating*," which included: setting and positioning; mood and atmosphere; participation, conversation, and encouragement; and time and pace of meal. Similarly, in March 2017, during a Health, Exercise and Nutrition for the Really Young (HENRY)[3] session that I attended at another children's centre in the borough, participants brainstormed some of the challenges they had encountered recently when feeding their children at home, and how they were trying to overcome them. Two of the five participants in the group mentioned that they were trying to reduce the time their children spent watching TV or looking at an iPad during mealtimes. For one of them, the solution was to turn their toddler's highchair towards the window, to distract them with what was happening outdoors.

Thus, it is perhaps unsurprising that Vivian shared these concerns with me, given the prominence that the eating environment receives in official discourse. In line with Lupton's notion that "experiential knowledge" about food and eating cannot be separated from biomedical understandings of nutrition (1996, 85), in these instances we can see that a circular process is taking place, by which biomedical discourse both *informs* and *is informed by* the social context in which it is developed. When it comes to the family meal, official discourse reinforces normative assumptions of what a 'civilised' and 'healthy' family eating environment might encompass.[4] As Murcott notes, a longstanding moral panic in the U.K. regarding the 'disappearance' of the family meal raises concerns about the perceived risk it poses to maintaining healthy diets, but is also linked to the fear that 'traditional' family life is disappearing (2000, 128).

Taking these questions of the family meal into consideration, Finch's notion of display (2007) is then relevant to understand what mothers shared with me in their accounts. Finch defines display as "the process by which individuals, and groups of individuals, convey to each other and to relevant audiences that certain of their actions…constitute 'doing family things'" (2007, 67). The concept of display differs from that of performance (or performativity) because the distinction between 'actor' and 'audience' is less distinct, since people's identities are constantly shifting between these two categories (ibid., 76). Using the example of a mother having a family meal at a restaurant, Finch explains how one can simultaneously be an actor and part of an audience: the mother behaves in a 'family-like' way for others, she observes how others at her table interact in 'family-like' ways, and imagines how her and her family members' actions will be interpreted as 'family-like' by other people at the restaurant (ibid.). I include these reflections since, as James and Curtis contend, different narratives that 'display family' highlight "not only *what* meanings people privately attribute to the concept of 'the family,' but also *how* these meanings interact with those dominant ideas of familialness" rooted "in the cultural and also political spheres of contemporary British life" (2010, 1164, original emphasis). As I explored in previous chapters, institutions – such as nurseries – also mediate and shape these notions of 'familialness.' Many of the aims women expressed about how they organised their foodwork, family meals, and how they hope their children's eating habits would develop, are very much linked to official and mainstream ideas of what a 'normal' family meal or diet should look like.

Thus, similarly to the importance Vivian gave to the eating environment, Rose emphasised eating together as a family in the two interviews that I conducted with her:

ROSE: *I'm trying, as they're getting older, what I'm trying to do is to get all of us eating together, because I believe that's really important. And when Susie was little I was really struggling with that because I felt like I was cooking something for the grownups and something for the children, but I'm trying now, increasingly, to cook something that all of us can eat together. I think a big issue with that is not to make things too hot and spicy. So I guess there's a difference between flavour and…spiciness. And I definitely think it's understandable that they're not going to like something spicy. I only started liking spicy food very recently, you know…but we are trying different flavours. So yeah I guess we try to make what we eat quite varied…and yeah, [to Susie] we try different things don't we? And I think you're not always sure if you haven't had something before.*

SUSIE: *Mhmmm… [nods]*

FV: *It sounds like eating together as a family is something that really matters to you…*

ROSE: *Yeah, it really does. And as I said, now that they're a bit older I'm finding that easier. I think when…the phase that I found particularly tricky was when Toby only just started to eat [solid] food. So obviously he would be eating really different to what Susie would be eating, and then [my husband and I] would probably be eating something different again, so I struggled with that, and also the time of the day…but now they're getting older. [To Susie] Quite often I will eat with you, won't I? If daddy is not around in the evening?*

SUSIE: *Or if you're not around in the evening, daddy eats with us!*

ROSE: *Yeah! Exactly. But that happens less [laughs]. But yeah, we've only just gradually started...if my husband can get back in time then we all eat together, and I think that's really nice and that's important. So I hope, increasingly, we can do that, and also that we can all eat the same thing, because I also believe you have everything on the table and everyone helps themselves, and that also encourages children, and they see that they're eating the same as grown-ups so...yeah I'm trying to do more of that.*

In Rose's account, a sense of responsibility not only for feeding her children healthy food, but also ensuring that the family eats together was evident, and was considered a priority even in instances when eating together (healthily) meant working double. During our follow-up interview, it surfaced that to fulfil this aim Rose was also willing to put aside some of her own food preferences to promote family unity and enact the values which were important to her. During our first encounter, she had told me that she did not eat meat for ethical reasons, but that she wanted Rose and Toby to eat meat until they could decide for themselves whether to eat it or not. In our second interview, she recounted a recent event that she was happy about:

ROSE: *I think something we've been doing more and more since we last saw you in August is trying to eat all of us together, and it's not always possible for my husband to be back in time, but when he can be, what we aim to do is to eat all of us together at six o'clock. And I feel like that's getting easier as they're getting a little older and we can pretty much all eat the same thing. But in terms of that role model thing, I think it's really important to have that family time, you know, so that we can all have a conversation and it's not like, ok the kids eat and then we eat later. And occasionally it happens, but more often than not we're all eating together, and what I'm also trying to do is having...sharing things, that I put out on the table and they see us helping ourselves, so as they get older they can help themselves and choose what they eat, all of that, that's important to have as a central tenet of family life.*

FV: *So that's a confidence building thing for the children as well?*

ROSE: *Yeah, I think so, I think so, and that that's a normal thing for them, that we eat all together and that's something we try to do. Something that we did recently, that we don't do often, is that we cooked a full Sunday lunch, because I don't eat meat, we don't tend to...you know, we would eat something together Sunday lunchtime, we don't have a roast, but [this time] we went to the butcher and bought some meat, and we had the roast potatoes, the Yorkshire pudding, you know, proper pudding, and vegetables... [to Susie] did you like that? When we had our Sunday lunch? Yeah it was quite nice wasn't it? And it's a funny thing, it does feel like there's more of a sense of occasion...and you know, it's not like I want to spend all of Sunday morning cooking, but actually that was quite a nice element to it as well...and it was good, wasn't it? So I don't know, there was something more to it than just all of us having pasta together. I think we'll probably try to do more of that, more often as well.*

What Rose shared with me echoes some of the deeply embedded notions about the centrality of the family meal, of eating together as a way of 'doing family' (Brannen, O'Connell, and Mooney 2013, 428), and perhaps a recognition that "contemporary families are defined more by 'doing' family things than by 'being' a family" (Finch 2007, 66). Lupton, similarly, puts forward that family meals are central to western imaginaries of *the* family, which also further contributes to the project of 'civilising' children (1996, 38).

Importantly, to Lupton "Any discussion of the role of food and eating in the context of the family must incorporate an analysis of the meanings and norms around motherhood and femininity" (1996, 38). Indeed, the link between 'good' food and 'good' parenting has already been emphasised, and the pressure women are particularly under to not be perceived as 'bad' parents because of their feeding practices has also been explored. Although it is important not to focus solely on the ways in which foodwork can function oppressively in mother's lives, it is also important to question how this unequal distribution of labour is reinforced by, and is reinforcing, traditional gender norms. As Cairns and Johnston have argued, viewing the individualistic approach to food and eating through the lens of gender is particularly urgent because it reveals that women's foodwork – and caring about the health of the family – is often simply considered to be women's *choice*, rather than a practice upheld by structural gender norms that promote the idea that foodwork is (by nature) women's work (2015, 13).

The responsibility women feel towards maintaining family unity through mealtimes came across quite vividly in some of the comments that participants made. The degree to which Vivian's partner shared her concern about creating an adequate eating environment for Fred, the importance Rose's husband attributed to eating together as a family, or Maria's father's commitment to 'eating healthily,' are unknown to me. However, participants seemed to experience these as issues they predominantly needed to take into their hands. Further, Rose's account of making the Sunday roast point to some of the tensions discussed by Cairns and Johnston. Rose described the meal as an overall pleasant and happy experience, but one which nonetheless also involved her forgoing part of the meal (since she does not eat meat) as well as having "*to spend all of Sunday morning cooking.*" Aside from the implications of managing these different tasks and expectations, what transpires in these narratives is also the importance of having (or not having) a sense of control over foodwork within the household, and beyond.

Being in control (ii): managing social relations

Like Rose and Vivian, a lack of agreement or synchronicity with partners on matters related to food was also voiced by Adriana, as well as a sense of having to put aside her own views about food. In our first interview, she told me:

When Maria eats ice-cream at school she's very happy. She says, 'Mummy, they gave me ice-cream, and you never want to give me any ice-cream'... and well, I don't like to give it to her, actually, but her father does [...] When she behaves well he will reward her that way, he will give her a sweet...and it's somewhat inevitable now, it's out of my hands. I try to reward her in other ways, I always tell her, 'If you behave we can watch a film, or we can go to the park,' but I never give her sweets or ice-cream as a reward...only her father [does].[5]

Out of all participants, Adriana was the one who shared the most insights regarding her husband's involvement in feeding their daughter. Her accounts of her husband's use of sweets as rewards are similar to some of Vivian's comments about her partner not being as concerned about Fred's screen time as she was. Nonetheless, as mentioned at the beginning of this chapter, this is a version of family life told from the perspective of my participants. What they might have experienced as a lack of cooperation from part of their male partners might have in fact have been intended as an act of care by fathers. Whilst foodwork might 'make mothers' in particular ways, it also works to blur other categories: in Adriana's and Vivian's accounts, fathers are almost infantilised, and seem to need to be guided in ways similar to their own children.

Managing social relations within the family, as part of wanting to maintain control of children's diets, also manifested itself in accounts about imbalances in the distribution of foodwork. This came up in conversation with Amanda, a second-generation West African woman who worked full time as a fitness instructor. In my notes from the interview, I recounted:

We talk about how there still seems to be a lot of responsibility placed on mothers to cook and feed children. She says that it is really hard, that even if she and her partner "are equal, both paying the same, he doesn't pay for me, I don't pay for him" and "he loves food and loves to cook" that "somehow at the end of a long day I am the one who ends up doing the cleaning, the cooking and getting Sean [two-years-old] from a playgroup" and that she "doesn't know how that happens" – notes from a semi-structured interview, February 2017.

Similarly, I asked Vivian about the distribution of foodwork between her and her partner:

FV: *You said earlier you're also mostly in charge of cooking and buying food.*
VIVIAN: *Yeah.*
FV: *Is that because you work less hours?*
VIVIAN: *I was thinking about that just before you came, I was wondering why that is... [my partner] can cook, and he's a great cook, he has a different repertoire and a very different way of doing things, but I love his*

> *food. I don't know...maybe I'm more controlling. I'm someone who's much more regular with her food, so I'm someone who wants to have three meals per day...maybe I'm just someone who steps in more than he does. I tend to be the one who is in charge of the money, who's in charge of the food...I think I'm just more controlling I guess [laughs].*

FV: *But then that's something that you see as separate from being a mum?*

VIVIAN: *Yes.*

FV: *And you enjoy it?*

VIVIAN: *Yes...sometimes, I enjoy it, I certainly enjoy food!*

Whether women needed to negotiate not seeing eye-to-eye with their partners on certain matters, or had to sacrifice their time, views, or preferences to promote 'good' habits and family unity, these instances show a particular way of 'doing gender' through foodwork that is informed by, and reproduces, hegemonic femininity. This way of 'doing gender' is also deeply linked to, and normalised by, a desire to be in control (e.g. Beagan et al. 2008) – like in Vivian's account above. This normalisation of gender roles, simultaneously, can seemingly obscure that gender is a factor that contributes to the way in which foodwork is structured within one's household.

Women's desire to be in control did not only manifest within the family home, but also in extended family circles as well as other social contexts. One theme that sometimes emerged in these conversations was the idea that their own mothers did not have the 'right' ideas about food and eating. During a focused group discussion carried out at Ladybird, Olga said:

> *If my mum comes over, she spoils [my daughter] with sweets, and crisps, and all those sugary drinks, and...even, we have those Polish drinks, maybe you've seen them in the shops [...] it will look healthy, because it's carrot, peach, orange, something...but, it's just full of sugar, it really has no nutrition in it. And people are bringing this to [my daughter] saying, "Oh I think this is good," and I'm like, this isn't good, it's different to those juices that children have when they start eating, you know? It's completely different, but they still bring it over.*

Vivian explained something similar during our interview:

> *When my mum comes over, Fred knows he can twist her arm and get treats... and ask for things that he knows if he asks me he knows he won't get. But it's also the generational shift, you know. Like one day she brought some cheese... 'La vache qui rit,' The Laughing Cow. And I didn't think much about it, but [my partner] said, "What's this, what's this doing in the fridge?" And he was really against it, because it's super processed cheese. And it got me looking at the ingredients, and I realised he had a point. And I realised afterwards...I really liked processed cheeses, and I had been brought up having them. And so I had to tell my mum, please don't buy those cheeses again. And she said,*

*why not? And I had to say, because they're really processed and I want to avoid getting him [Fred] into processed foods. And she said...but all cheese is processed! And I didn't really have an argument for it...because all cheese kind of **is** processed...but she didn't really see anything wrong with it.*

Participants also expressed discomfort and frustration with some of the encounters they had with friends of theirs, both those that also have children and those that do not. Below is another extract from my notes from the conversation with Amanda:

Amanda narrates an episode from a picnic she had with some of her friends that also have children, and how she brought some home-made food to share with them. She tells me that her friends at some point asked her if it was ok to give Sean some cake they brought and she said yes, but then when she looked over she saw that they were opening a packet of store-bought cake, so she "ran over" and told them not to give it to Sean. She says that she could tell her friends got a bit offended ("as if I was saying that it [the cake] wasn't good enough for Sean") and that she felt bad, but that she didn't want him to eat that. She says, "So you see, even among friends it's hard." She tells me that when they saw her opening a Tupperware for Sean with broccoli in it they told her, sarcastically, "good luck with that." She justifies her behaviour that day by explaining her fear that once children discover and learn how to recognise certain (bad) foods they will then ask for them again.

Amanda's description of the picnic with her friends also points to what Faircloth (2014), drawing on Hays (1996), has identified as 'intensive parenting.' Because parenting – and feeding – are deeply tied to identity (Faircloth 2014, 47), parents' practices can function as a form of 'ideological work': by following certain parenting 'styles' mothers morally position themselves in relation to one another (ibid.). In Amanda's account, this tension is evident: the store-bought cake ('bad' food) and the box of broccoli ('good' food) were strong markers that defined what 'good' versus 'bad' parenting represented in this context. Parental accountability is thus a salient trope in these participants' narratives, but so is a concern that children will not be able to make the 'right' choices in the future if they are not taught what these choices are from an early age. This again points to the assumption that individual choice is a main determinant of health, which undermines that other material, structural, and social circumstances have an impact on children's eating.

Thus, whilst linked to them, many of the anxieties and frustrations expressed in these accounts are often ignored in nutritionist-driven approaches. In this understanding of food and eating, the social and moral values attached to food can be overlooked – unless they are attached to normative ideas of what constitutes a family meal. The socio-economic circumstances that determine people's diets, beyond biomedical understandings of what healthy eating means to them, are also often missing in this paradigm (e.g. Guthman 2014; Hayes-Conroy et al. 2014). As discussed in the previous chapter, these models, which tend to emphasise individual accountability for dietary intake (Lupton 1996, 72; Ulijaszek and McLennan 2016), also feed into the discourse of parental blame if children eat 'bad' foods (Maher, Fraser, and Lindsay 2010; Maher, Fraser, and Wright 2010; O'Connell and Brannen 2016; Harman, Faircloth, and Cappellini 2019). In this framing of the issue, the different contexts and social relations that children encounter as they develop their own habits and preferences are often also not taken into consideration. Parents are not the only people in charge of determining their children's diets, especially as they grow older and they become more exposed to media and advertising from the food industry (Martens, Southerton, and Scott 2004, 166).

Further, other relatives, adults outside of the family, as well as peers, also influence children's food intake. The impact other people have on children's eating, aside from their parents, is explored by Albon (2007) in a paper on using food-maps as a tool to track families' eating patterns. Food-maps, she argues, are a visual representation of the (often) vast array of people, relationships, and places that can affect children's (and adults') diets (2007, 257). Although she suggests this method can be used by health and early years professionals "involved in making a positive impact on people's diets" (ibid., 245), and thus links to a more nutrition-driven approach to food and eating, it nonetheless brings to the fore the complex web of social relations and settings that children engage with, and which influence their diets – as also suggested by the accounts of my participants.

Children's encounters outside the home were often described by mothers as an interference to their sense of having control over their children's diets and budding preferences, and were thus often described to me as a source of anxiety. Thus, it is also important to consider how negotiations between parents and children are shaped by the experiences children have outside the home and with other people, and the implications this can have for how we think about children's agency. In the next section, I return to Bakhtin's work on the 'dialogic' (1986), introduced in Chapter 4, to explore the idea that children and parents co-produce knowledge and practices, rather than simply engaging in a power struggle.

Food and the dialogic (ii): Bakhtin at the intersection of the home and school environments

Above, I introduced Faircloth's (2014) discussion of 'intensive motherhood,' prevalent in many Euro-American contexts. She contends that this is based on an emotionally and energy consuming "belief that a child's needs must be put first and that mothering should be child-centred" (2014, 26). Faircloth claims that this has important implications for mothers' identities, as intensive parenting (with all its varying manifestations) "remains an important 'cultural script' or 'ideal' to which parents respond in negotiating their own practices" (ibid., 31).

Much of the literature that deals with intensive parenting tends to emphasise the deferential role of mothers. Miller's famous example of how "infants grow mothers" in North London (1997) delves into this topic. He concludes that, despite women's best efforts to promote a 'natural,' 'organic' diet for their children, they ultimately experience motherhood as a series of 'defeats' as children develop their own preferences later in life (1997, 74–75). Meanwhile, in trying to be ideal mothers, he argues, women "allow the infant to represent the complete negation of their previous life project" (ibid., 72). The parallel between feeding children 'good food' and being a 'good mother' has already been emphasised. I have assessed how this assumption can act oppressively in women's lives, including the imbalance in the distribution of foodwork between men and women. This is evidenced in the literature I have examined in this chapter (e.g. DeVault 1991; Cairns and Johnston 2015; Harman, Faircloth, and Cappellini 2019), but also in some of my participants' accounts, who, at times, described putting their own needs aside in the pursuit of providing their children the food they deemed healthy, or when maintaining family unity through mealtimes.

However, I would now like to shift the emphasis in this discussion by drawing again from Bakhtin's work on the dialogic, to argue that mothers and children are 'becoming' in relation to one another in a mutualistic, rather than a unidirectional, way. Albon and Rosen have suggested that Bakhtinian theory sheds light on how individual selves create meaningful knowledge through dialogic relationships with others (2014, 9). Writing specifically about young children's eating practices, White (2017) has argued that mealtimes offer children an opportunity to negotiate and test different norms and meanings acquired from the adult world, rather than always contesting these.

Whilst participants spoke to me about the challenges they encountered as their children grew in their independence, children's expanding knowledge(s) and practices cannot only be conceived of as 'defeats' for their mothers, as suggested in some of the literature. Indeed, when at school, children also reproduced some of the norms and practices that their mothers promoted at home. Conversely, some of the practices children brought from the school into the home might have been well-received by parents. In my notes after the home interview I conducted with Rose, I wrote:

> During our interview today, Susie and Toby wanted Rose's attention a couple of times, asking for food: "I'm talking to Fran right now so I can't cut you up watermelon right now, you can have it for supper," she said to Toby mid-sentence shortly after our conversation began. Susie asked for a clementine and, like Toby, was asked to wait until the interview was finished. After we were done talking and I was getting ready to leave, Susie reiterated her request for a clementine, to which Rose agreed. Whilst Rose peeled the fruit, Susie asked: "But cut them up like at Ladybird!"

Rose expressed her approval for the ways in which staff encouraged children to eat fruit and vegetables at Ladybird, such as cutting up clementines in the distinct way that Susie seemed to like. Returning to Corsaro's notion of 'interpretive reproduction' (2011), trying to understand children's viewpoints also involves understanding what they deem meaningful about their everyday lives. And, whilst at times this might mean that children contest adult norms, some of what gets appropriated and reinterpreted by them can also meet adults' objectives, as discussed in Chapters 3 and 4.

Some of the details that emerge from the ethnographic and child-centred research that I conducted at Ladybird is evidence of this. During a photo-elicitation activity I carried out with Maria, Adriana's daughter, she echoed some of the views that Adriana shared with me during our interviews some months later. As she flipped through different stock images from the box I used for the activity, Maria stopped to look at a photo of a group of children eating pizza out of a take-away box. As I did for each image that the children chose during this activity, I asked Maria what she thought was happening in the picture; "*They're eating pizza!*" she said. "*And do you like pizza?*" I asked. She responded: "*Yes! And my brother buys pizza, but then my mum says, 'No more pizza!' to him. Because pizza is also a golosina [Spanish word for a candy or sweet treat].*"[6] I thought Maria's choice of word to describe pizza was interesting – perhaps anything that she considered 'unhealthy' was a sweet in her vocabulary. Her use of this term became clearer to me in the conversations I later had with her mother Adriana, who spoke a lot about her dislike of *golosinas,* especially when she referred to her husband's and son's diets, which she considered unhealthy.

Several times, Maria referred to the South American cuisine her family made with fondness. During the same photo-elicitation activity, she also chose to talk about an image showing a group of children in a nursery setting helping themselves to pieces of bread from a plate in front of them. When other children came across this photo they would often make generic comments about their experiences at tea-club or lunchtime, or say that it was one of them or their friends eating at Ladybird (even if all the photos I used for the activity were stock images). When I asked Maria what she thought was happening in the photo she told me that the children were eating *empanadas.*[7] Maria told me she liked *empandas* very much, and shared her experience about a day on which her mother was making *empanadas* at home and burnt her hand, so her father had to learn to cook this dish while her mother recovered from the burn. I thought Maria's comments during the photo-elicitation activity were an interesting way for her to insert her home environment into a depiction of school: *empanadas* are an emblematic Latin American dish, and which would not have been served as a meal at Ladybird.

Imagining a well-liked dish outside of the home environment is indicative of the role children (particularly migrant children or children of migrants) can play in the reproduction of foodways, culture, and culinary traditions, as several scholars have noted (see for example Janowski 2012; Bajic-Hajdukovic 2013). However, it also suggests, again, that what makes food valuable for children (as well as adults) is the convivial dimension of mealtimes: sharing favourite dishes was often a way for children to express care in role-play, for example, as I have also shown in Chapter 4. Yet, not only was food an important channel through which children fostered peer group unity, it was also (like in Maria's case) a medium through which self-identity can be expressed. As Clark contends for the case of understanding children's spaces, children are very aware of how their lived environment relates to other people, things, and places that in turn relate to themselves (2010, 80). By the same token, I argue that examining children's relationship to food is a productive

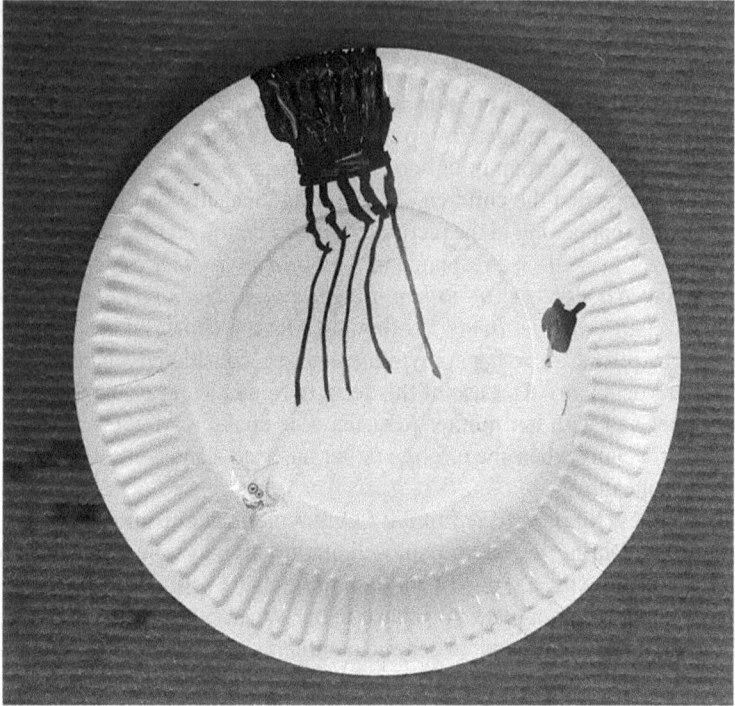

Figure 6.1 "Spaghetti, and a special fork for my little brother" – Susie (4).
Photograph by the author.

way of understanding their relationship with the wide array of categories that makes up their sense of self and social belonging.

For example, the importance Rose afforded to eating together as a family was evident when Susie took part in an activity in which I asked children to draw their favourite foods to have at home on a paper plate. Susie made the picture shown in Figure 6.1.

When I asked Susie what was in the drawing, she explained that it was, *"Spaghetti and a special fork for my little brother."* Hearing Rose's views about family meals during our home interviews a few months later gave further meaning to Susie's drawing, explaining why she might have chosen to depict an element that also included her little brother in it. During one of our interviews, Rose said:

> *It's nice for them [Susie and Toby] to eat together, and now they can also eat the same thing...which I think they both enjoy, and they have an impact on each other. Equally that's also why I think it's important for me to eat with them...sometimes I'll cook them something different, but most times we'll just have the same things [...] even if children are just eating together I think it's nice, it's companionable isn't it?*

As shown throughout this chapter, threaded through mothers' narratives was the sense that foodwork is not only important because it sustains the health and integrity of one's family, but also because, through it, each woman taught their children things that mattered to them. We have already seen that for Adriana, Rose, Vivian, and Amanda, as well as most (if not all) parents I spoke to, teaching their children to eat healthily is a central priority, and eating together as a family is seen as a moment to teach one's children about care and conviviality. Whilst mothers communicated their deep concern for a variety of factors that might negatively influence their children, as well as worry that their own feeding practices were not sufficiently 'good,' what children spoke about during the activities we did together at Ladybird suggest that some of the norms and practices that mothers were so eager to promote were indeed also meaningful to their children.

Yet, this was often unknown to them – parents were curious to find out what and how their sons and daughters ate at school, so asked me about it, and were pleasantly surprised when I related some of these anecdotes to them. Equally, children brought some of the things they considered valuable from the school environment into the home, which parents also seemed to approve of, like Susie's request for fruit to be cut up in a certain way, or Fred's retelling of how we had 'lettuce competitions' at tea-club, which Vivian embraced as an idea to encourage him to eat vegetables at home. Whilst these might be considered examples that indicate how an 'intensive mothering' culture is enacted in the everyday lives of children and parents, it also emphasises that children and mothers 'make each other' in a much more mutualistic and creative way. Following Bakhtin, Mayerfeld Bell suggests that a 'dialogic conception of culture' is a useful way to examine how culture moves from one generation to the next, and to both understand cultural change as well as resistance to cultural change (1998, 59). He contends that:

> *Taking into account the words of others is the principal phenomenological requirement of dialogic interaction.* In a conversation, we do not say just anything about anything. We negotiate, we discuss, we mistake, we mislead, and we otherwise stumble to a jointly creative response to the conditions of our understandings and misunderstandings.
>
> (ibid., 63, original emphasis)

The interactions I have described – both those that happened between mothers and children together, and those that happened with children and I at Ladybird – mirror Mayerfeld Bell's conceptualisation of culture as dialogic, as "an interactive experience of difference and sameness" through which we all negotiate knowledge(s) and practices in relation to one another (ibid., 62), both when we are together and apart.

Furthermore, a Bakhtinian perspective can also be a useful alternative lens with which to think about power relations, as mentioned above. In previous chapters as well as here, I have drawn from Foucault to emphasise that governmentality is enacted on children and parents via the state, institutions, between individuals, and through self-surveillance (Foucault 1988; Lupton 1995). This process, as several scholars have argued, has particularly intensified in advanced liberal democracies such as Britain's (e.g. Rose 1996; Moss and Petrie 2000; Mitchell 2014), which are organised around the premise that society is populated by autonomous, rational, self-regulating, and self-improving individuals (Mitchell 2014, 12). However, by turning to Bakhtin, some of the elements inherent to that process of governmentality, and individualisation, can be challenged. Examining the 'back and forth' interaction between the different realms within which discourses and practices about children's food emerge reveals the 'non-linearity' of feeding and eating. Examining dialogic processes sheds light on the messiness and unpredictability of everyday life, of caring through food, and the 'open-endedness' of caring relations (Mol 2008, 18).

In this chapter, for example, having highlighted how children bring some of the practices that emerged at Ladybird into their homes shows that children's and parents' practices are not simply shaped and constrained by discourses that are happening at a macro-level. Some of the norms and behaviours that children created (and co-created) within Ladybird's micro-context (also drawing from the other social worlds they inhabit, like their home environments) serve very different purposes to those advocated in official discourse. The repetitive, playful, and caring practices that children engaged in at school emphasised the convivial and pleasurable dimension of eating together. This goes against the individualistic, nutrition-driven approach advocated in official discourse and, by momentarily empathising or entering children's points of view, adults could also challenge these overarching narratives (Marjanovic-Shane and White 2014; White 2014).

This framework can be particularly useful to explore the micro-level interactions in the home and school environment, in which these creative, co-productive, and relational interactions can be given more attention and consideration than on a macro- or policy-level. It can also not only challenge the nutrition-driven approaches to food and eating that I have critiqued throughout this book, but also the rhetoric of parental blame attached to these, which has a particularly negative impact on mothers, as I have shown. Importantly, it can also help us think further about children's agentic role in the reproduction of norms and behaviours. As Corsaro has argued, the notion of interpretive reproduction offers a vision of children's development as collectively produced with others throughout the life course (2005, 231). To Corsaro, recognising children's participation in cultural (re) production, both in their peer groups and with adults, is a way to "bridge the micro-macro gap" (ibid., 232). And, as I have shown, this crossing over of contexts helps us to examine the particular, and to challenge universal narratives about feeding and eating practices within institutions and households.

If we think of children and mothers as engaged in a more mutualistic, collective, and relational process of becoming – together – then we might also rethink (and challenge) some of the macro-scale narratives about feeding children, and children's eating. Whilst official and mainstream understandings of parents' roles in teaching their children about food are largely unidirectional, by exploring how children bring their daily experiences outside of the household into the home environment (and vice-versa), adults and children are involved in a much more collaborative project of becoming in relation to one another. By paying attention to the social value of food, and emphasising how fundamental it is to children's and adults' sense of self and belonging, universal (official) narratives about food and eating can be challenged.

Notes

1 Adriana is from Latin America. This interview was conducted in Spanish; the translation is my own.
2 Own translation from Spanish.
3 'The HENRY Approach to Preventing Childhood Obesity' was introduced and discussed in detail in Chapter 1.
4 See Elliott and Hore (2016) for a discourse analysis of food, youth, and morality in the U.K., for example; whilst the emphasis of their study is policy discourse about school meals, they emphasise how notions about 'family values' are repeatedly deployed to make claims about the kind of habits children should be encouraged to develop.
5 Own translation from Spanish.
6 Own translation from Spanish.
7 "Empanada, a baked or fried pastry stuffed with meat, cheese, vegetables, fruits, and other ingredients. Empanadas can be found around the world, especially in Latin America, Spain, and Portugal" (*Britannica Academic*, s.v. "Empanada," accessed January 29, 2019, https://academic.eb.com/levels/collegiate/article/empanada/626875).

References

Afflerback, Sara, Shannon K. Carter, Amanda Koontz Anthony, and Liz Grauerholz. 2013. 'Infant-Feeding Consumerism in the Age of Intensive Mothering and Risk Society'. *Journal of Consumer Culture* 13 (3): 387–405. https://doi.org/10.1177/1469540513485271.

Albon, Deborah. 2007. 'Exploring Food and Eating Patterns Using Food-Maps'. *Nutrition & Food Science* 37 (4): 254–59. https://doi.org/10.1108/00346650710774622.

———. 2015. 'Nutritionally "Empty" but Full of Meanings: The Socio-Cultural Significance of Birthday Cakes in Four Early Childhood Settings'. *Journal of Early Childhood Research* 13 (1): 79–92.

Albon, Deborah, and Rachel Rosen. 2014. *Negotiating Adult-Child Relationships in Early Childhood Research*. London: Routlegde.

Allen, Patricia, and Carolyn Sachs. 2012. 'Women and Food Chains: The Gendered Politics of Food'. In *Taking Food Public: Redefining Foodways in a Changing World*, edited by Psyche Williams Forson and Carole Counihan, 23–40. New York: Taylor and Francis.

Allison, Anne. 1991. 'Japanese Mothers and Obentōs: The Lunch-Box as Ideological State Apparatus'. *Anthropological Quarterly* 64 (4): 195–208. https://doi.org/10.2307/3317212.

Bajic-Hajdukovic, Ivana. 2013. 'Food, Family, and Memory: Belgrade Mothers and Their Migrant Children'. *Food and Foodways* 21 (1): 46–65. https://doi.org/10.1080/0740971 0.2013.764787.

Bakhtin, Mikhail. 1986. *Speech Genres and Other Late Essays*. Austin: University of Texas Press.

Beagan, Brenda, Gwen E. Chapman, Andrea D'Sylva, and B. Raewyn Bassett. 2008. '"It's Just Easier for Me to Do It": Rationalizing the Family Division of Foodwork'. *Sociology* 42 (4): 653–71. https://doi.org/10.1177/0038038508091621.

Boni, Zofia. 2019. '"My Mum Feeds Me, but Really, I Eat Whatever I Want!": A Relational Approach to Feeding and Eating'. In *Feeding Children Inside and Outside the Home*, edited by Vicki Harman, Benedetta Cappellini, and Charlotte Faircloth, 107–123. Abingdon: Routledge.

———. 2023. *Feeding Anxieties: The Politics of Children's Food in Poland*. Vol. 6. New Anthropologies of Europe: Perspectives and Provocations. New York and Oxford: Berghahn Books.

Brannen, Julia, Rebecca O'Connell, and Ann Mooney. 2013. 'Families, Meals and Synchronicity: Eating Together in British Dual Earner Families'. *Community, Work & Family* 16 (4): 417–34. https://doi.org/10.1080/13668803.2013.776514.

Cairns, Kate, and Josée Johnston. 2015. *Food and Femininity*. New York: Bloomsbury.

Corsaro, William. 2005. 'Collective Action and Agency in Young Children's Peer Culture'. In *Studies in Modern Childhood: Society, Agency, Culture*, edited by Jens Qvortrup, 231–47. Basingstoke: Palgrave Macmillan.

———. 2011. *The Sociology of Childhood*. London: SAGE Publications.

DeVault, Marjorie. 1991. *Feeding the Family: The Social Organization of Caring as Gendered Work*. Chicago: University of Chicago Press.

Elliott, Sinikka, and Sarah Bowen. 2018. 'Defending Motherhood: Morality, Responsibility, and Double Binds in Feeding Children'. *Journal of Marriage and Family* 80 (2): 499–520. https://doi.org/10.1111/jomf.12465.

Elliott, Victoria, and Beth Hore. 2016. '"Right Nutrition, Right Values": The Construction of Food, Youth and Morality in the UK Government 2010–2014'. *Cambridge Journal of Education* 46 (2): 177–93. https://doi.org/10.1080/0305764X.2016.1158785.

Faircloth, Charlotte. 2014. 'Intensive Parenting and the Expansion of Parenting'. In *Parenting Culture Studies*, edited by Ellie Lee, Jennie Bristow, Charlotte Faircloth, and Jan Macvarish, 25–50. Basingstoke: Palgrave Macmillan.

Faircloth, Charlotte, and Marjorie Murray. 2015. 'Parenting: Kinship, Expertise, and Anxiety'. *Journal of Family Issues* 36 (9): 1115–29.Finch, Janet. 2007. 'Displaying Families.' *Sociology* 41 (1): 65–81.

Foucault, Michel. 1988. 'Technologies of the Self'. In *Technologies of the Self : A Seminar with Michel Foucault*, edited by Luther H. Martin, Huck Gutman, and Patrick H. Hutton, 16. London: Tavistock Publications Ltd.

———. 1991. 'Governmentality'. In *The Foucault Effect: Studies in Governmentality, with Two Lectures by and an Interview with Michel Foucault*, edited by Graham Burchell, Colin Gordon, and Peter Miller, 87–104. Chicago: University of Chicago Press.

Guthman, Julie. 2014. 'Introducing Critical Nutrition: A Special Issue on Dietary Advice and Its Discontents'. *Gastronomica: The Journal of Critical Food Studies* 14 (3): 1–4.

Harman, Vicki, Charlotte Faircloth, and Benedetta Cappellini. 2019. 'Introduction'. In *Feeding Children Inside and Outside the Home: Critical Perspectives*, edited by Vicki Harman, Benedetta Cappellini, and Charlotte Faircloth, 1–7. Abingdon: Routledge.

Hays, Sharon. 1996. *The Cultural Contradictions of Motherhood*. New Haven: Yale University Press.

Hayes-Conroy, Jessica, Adele Hite, Kendra Klein, Charlotte Biltekoff, and Aya H. Kimura. 2014. 'Doing Nutrition Differently'. *Gastronomica: The Journal of Critical Food Studies* 14 (3): 56–66.

James, Allison, and Penny Curtis. 2010. 'Family Displays and Personal Lives'. *Sociology* 44 (6): 1163–80. https://doi.org/10.1177/0038038510381612.

Janowski, Monica. 2012. 'Introduction: Consuming Memories of Home in Constructing the Present and Imagining the Future'. *Food and Foodways* 20 (3–4): 175–86. https://doi.org/10.1080/07409710.2012.715960.

Lee, Ellie, Jennie Bristow, Charlotte Faircloth, and Jan Macvarish. 2014. Parenting Culture Studies. London: Palgrave Macmillan.

Lupton, Deborah. 1995. *The Imperative of Health: Public Health and the Regulated Body.* London: SAGE Publications.

———. 1996. *Food, the Body and the Self.* London: SAGE Publications.

———. 2012. 'Infant Embodiment and Interembodiment: A Review of Sociocultural Perspectives'. *Childhood* 20 (1): 37–50.

Maher, JaneMaree, Suzanne Fraser, and Jo Lindsay. 2010. 'Between Provisioning and Consuming?: Children, Mothers and "Childhood Obesity"'. *Health Sociology Review* 19 (3): 304–16.

Maher, JaneMaree, Suzanne Fraser, and Jan Wright. 2010. 'Framing the Mother: Childhood Obesity, Maternal Responsibility and Care'. *Journal of Gender Studies* 19 (3): 233–47. https://doi.org/10.1080/09589231003696037.

Marjanovic-Shane, Ana, and E. Jayne White. 2014. 'When the Footlights Are Off: A Bakhtinian Interrogation of Play as Postupok'. *International Journal of Play* 3 (2): 119–35. https://doi.org/10.1080/21594937.2014.931686.

Martens, Lydia, Dale Southerton, and Sue Scott. 2004. 'Bringing Children (and Parents) into the Sociology of Consumption towards a Theoretical and Empirical Agenda'. *Journal of Consumer Culture* 4 (2): 155–82.

Mayerfeld Bell, Michael. 1998. 'Culture as Dialogue'. In *Bakhtin and the Human Sciences: No Last Words*, edited by Michael Mayerfeld Bell and Michael Gardiner, 49–62. London: SAGE Publications.

Mitchell, Dean. 2014. *Governmentality: Power and Rule in Modern Society.* London: SAGE Publications.

Mol, Annemarie. 2008. *The Logic of Care: Health and the Problem of Patient Choice.* London: Routledge.

Moss, Peter, and Pat Petrie. 2000. *From Children's Services to Children's Spaces.* London: Routledge/Falmer.

Murcott, Anne. 2000. 'Understanding Life-Style and Food Use: Contributions from the Social Sciences'. *British Medical Bulletin* 56 (1): 121–32.

O'Connell, Rebecca, and Julia Brannen. 2014. 'Children's Food, Power and Control: Negotiations in Families with Younger Children in England'. *Childhood* 2 (1): 87–102.

O'Connell, Rebecca, and Julia Brannen. 2016. *Food, Families and Work.* London: Bloomsbury.

Rose, Nikolas. 1996. 'Governing "Advanced" Liberal Democracies'. In *Foucault and Political Reason. Liberalism, Neo-Liberalism and Rationalities of Government*, edited by Andrew Barry, Thomas Osborne, and Nikolas Rose, 37–64. London: Routledge.

Ulijaszek, Stanley J., and Amy K. McLennan. 2016. 'Framing Obesity in UK Policy from the Blair Years, 1997–2015: The Persistence of Individualistic Approaches despite Overwhelming Evidence of Societal and Economic Factors, and the Need for Collective Responsibility'. *Obesity Reviews* 17 (5): 397–411. https://doi.org/10.1111/obr.12386.

White, E. Jayne. 2017. 'A Feast of Fools: Mealtimes as Democratic Acts of Resistance and Collusion in Early Childhood Education'. *Knowledge Cultures* 5 (3): 85. https://doi.org/10.22381/KC5320177.

White, Elizabeth Jayne. 2014. 'Are You "Avin a Laff?": A Pedagogical Response to Bakhtinian Carnivalesque in Early Childhood Education'. *Educational Philosophy and Theory* 46 (8): 898–913. https://doi.org/10.1080/00131857.2013.781497.s

Conclusion

Three endings

July 2017:

The 'tea-clubbers' and some of the staff have prepared a special send off for me on the last session of tea-club. The tablecloth has been sprinkled with shiny confetti and, among the usual snacks consisting of fruit and vegetables, there are also plates filled with crisps on the table today – 'treats' for a special occasion. After I take my seat, Crystal and Tommy emerge from the kitchen (usually a space off limits to them) carrying a heart-shaped vanilla sponge cake that the children helped decorate using icing of different colours. The words on the cake read: "We'll miss you Fran!" Adam hands me a big envelope with a card that the staff and children have made for me. While I read my card, Crystal asks me, with her usual confident demeanour, if I want to drink water or juice (another 'treat' today) and pours me some water from the jug after I state my preference. She passes me the snack plates with carrot sticks and sliced apples, and also tells me I can only take five crisps, following Ruby's instructions that each person can only eat five crips. We eat together, then play some of the usual tea-club games, and make cards for each other as keepsakes.

The last session of tea-club was an emotional one for me. Although I still spent a few more weeks volunteering at the children's centre after the school year ended, most of the children who I got to know well over the year that I spent at Ladybird Nursery and Children's Centre I would not see again, except during home interviews in some cases. Aside from three-year-old Fred, those sitting at the table with me that day (Tommy, Crystal, Susie, Adam, and Gerry) were going to 'big school' in September. I wondered what kind of mealtime set-ups they would encounter in their respective new schools, and the type of interactions that would unfold while they sat with their future peers to eat together. Based on Ruby's accounts of her past jobs (examined in Chapter 3), and the things she tried to teach to the children in preparation for the start of primary education, I imagined more restricted (and restrictive) experiences lied ahead of them.

Nonetheless, while we ate our snacks and supper together for one last time that summer, the same interactions that I had observed and become familiar with during

DOI: 10.4324/9781003297642-8

the 11 months I had spent at Ladybird repeated themselves. Crystal showed her caring character by offering me drinks and food, the rest of the group confidently helped themselves to the food they wanted (and sneakily overlooked Ruby's instructions that they each only eat five crisps), and they recognised the significance of that day's occasion, marked by the cake, crisps, and juice – special treats that we would not otherwise have had during a regular tea-club afternoon. Many of the playful and humorous interactions that had also become part of our routine took place during the session. That afternoon, I got a final glimpse into how interpretive reproduction (Corsaro 2011) happened in practice among this group of children. I sswas reminded of the various means by which they made mealtimes meaningful for themselves, at times subverting adults' control. And again, a recurrent contradiction emerged: that food, even – or perhaps especially – 'unhealthy' food, is very commonly used to show and express care, by children and adults alike.

July 2017:

It is the last day of school and the main hallway at Ladybird is buzzing with activity. To mark the end of the school year, the school is hosting an 'International Food Summer Party.' Two long tables have been set up in the hallway, which families have filled up with dozens of home-made dishes: this fragrant assortment of savoury and

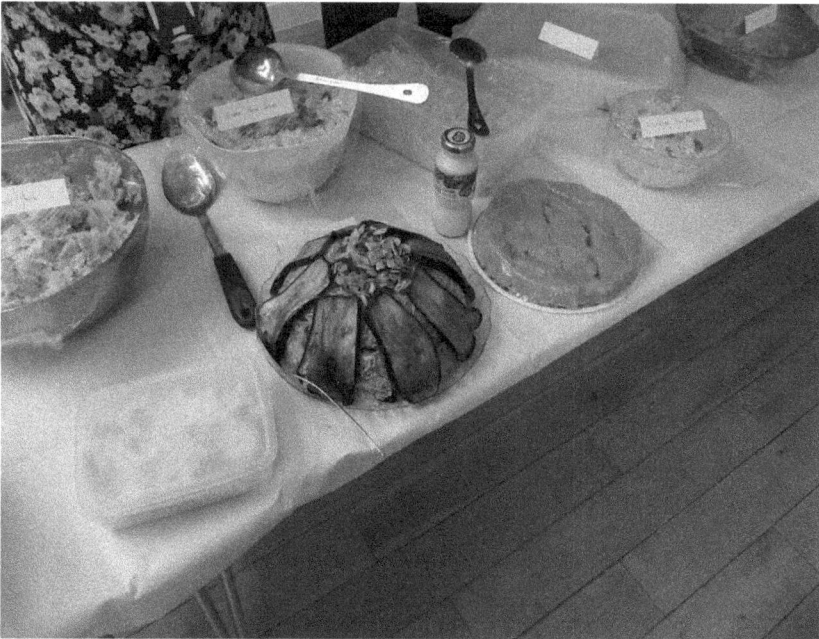

Figure 7.1 Home-made dishes made at the 'International Food Summer Party' at Ladybird Nursery and Children's Centre.

Photograph by the author.

sweet foods is a testament to the diversity of the school's student body. I read the lit-
tle cards on which parents were asked by staff to write the name of each dish (and
to indicate whether there are any allergens in the food). There is West African Jollof
rice and jerk chicken, a cous-cous salad made by an Algerian family, Indian onion
bhajis, a Vietnamese mango and banana steamed cake with coconut cream. There
are also more 'mainstream' dishes that have likely little to do with the cultural or eth-
nic background of the families who brought them: I spot several kinds of pasta plat-
ters (tomato pasta, 'Greek pasta salad,' tuna pasta), cucumber sandwiches, coleslaw
with raisins, scones with strawberry jam. Some store-bought foods are also included
in this mix: cocktail sausages, various dips next to carrots and celery sticks, olives,
and some 'healthy' crisps and crackers. Inside the children's centre (and eventually
behind a closed door) a small table has been set aside, where crisps, breadsticks,
fizzy drinks, chocolates, biscuits, and store-bought cakes [Figure 7.2] are placed.
This would be the only food left over after the party, which was then stored in the
staff common room and consumed in the coming days by the school staff.

In the couple of weeks leading up to this event, a sign-up sheet had been hanging
on one of the noticeboards at the school, on which parents were asked to write what
they would bring to the party ("*It can be a main dish, snack, dessert, or drink,*" the
instructions read). Joyce (the lead early years practitioner at the children's centre)

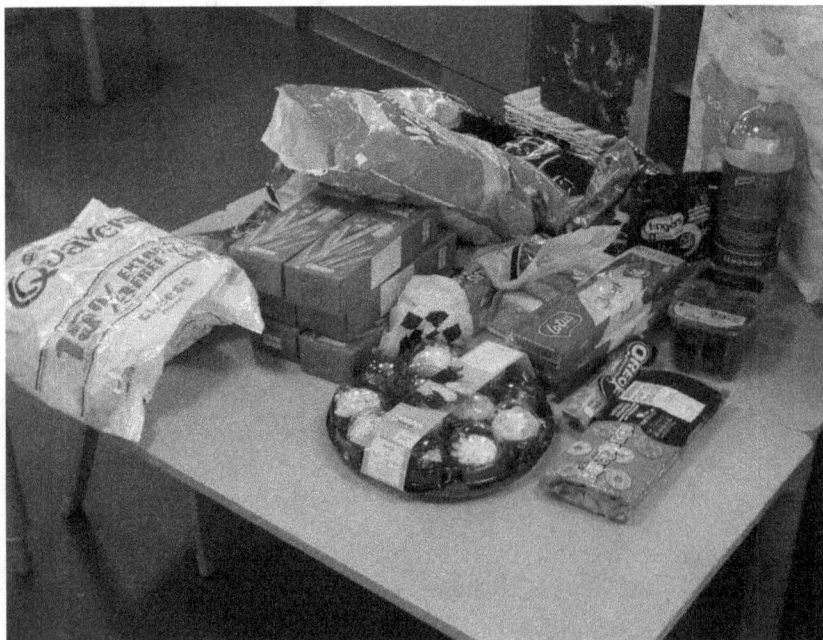

Figure 7.2 Store-bought foods and fizzy drinks not included in the 'International Food
          Summer Party' buffet.

Photograph by the author.

had told me she was worried that some families who were struggling financially might not come to the party if they could not contribute to the event with food or a drink. In the weeks leading up to the event, I heard her telling some of the parents on several occasions that it was OK if they were able to just bring a single portion of any dish, or a small snack, reassuring them that *"there will be plenty of food anyway."* Unlike other special events on which families were asked to bring food to share with the school community (such as Christmas), this time no special request had been made to not bring any store-bought or packaged foods, or fizzy drinks, to the party. I was therefore surprised when these items were relegated to a separate section of the school on the day of the event, a reminder of their abject position in official and mainstream discourses about food and eating.

Whilst it was not just families who were struggling financially that brought these foods – some were working parents who might have faced time constraints, for example – a few were those who lived in temporary accommodation, who might not have had adequate cooking facilities or food storage boxes to transport home-made dishes to the school, or indeed were those whom were relying on benefits to get by. Whilst the school staff tried to make this event inclusive to all, the way in which food contributions were laid out on the day of the party reflected some of the wider tensions about food and parenting that I had observed over the course of my fieldwork. The discordance between the universalism of policy and the particularism of feeding and eating was poignantly clear in this instance: policy and mainstream definitions of 'healthy food' excluded some families' expressions of care and conviviality on the day of the party.

November 2017:
 Joyce and her husband are moving back to their home country, as their work visas are expiring, and I have been invited to attend her leaving drinks alongside some of the other staff from Ladybird. It's been three months since the end of my fieldwork, so I'm looking forward to catching up with everyone and hearing how things are going at the nursery. I am surprised to find out that, of the group of five who are here tonight, there is just one teacher still working at Ladybird. The other two teachers and one early years practitioner have all moved on to other settings; all of them say the main reason for leaving was the strained relationship they had with the headteacher, a tension that I was aware of superficially, but that I never enquired people about during fieldwork. Aside from the early years practitioner, who now works at another children's centre in a nearby borough, all the others are now working in private settings. Emily, one of the teachers who had been working at Ladybird for almost 20 years, says that the nursery where she now works is a bit more 'standardized,' but that the pay is better. The others don't go into detail about their new jobs, rather reiterating how much happier they are working under a different manager, and affectionately mock their former colleague who is 'stuck' working at Ladybird. The conversation soon moves to other topics, as the rounds of drinks multiply and the evening carries on.

After this get-together, I reflected on an apparent pattern happening at Ladybird. During the second half of my fieldwork, several of the teachers and other staff (including lunch assistants) had been talking about looking for new jobs in other settings, about leaving Ladybird to retrain, or to pursue further education. Cynthia, one of the nursery teachers, had left in spring 2017 to begin a postgraduate degree. Another teacher, Brenda, resigned unexpectedly shortly after Cynthia left, explaining she felt burnt out, and was increasingly sceptical about the kind (and amount) of assessment of children's abilities she was required to do, which did not align with her training and vision of what nursery education should be like. I also knew of Robert's evening degree, and the new profession he fully transitioned to at the end of 2017. In December that year, he sent me a text-message in which he expressed his excitement at leaving his role as Ladybird's extended services manager. Robert had always been quite open with me about the negative direction he perceived the state-maintained early years sector to be heading towards, and the added pressure he faced (on top of his regular, main duties) because of the constant need to audit the activities and 'outcomes' at the children's centre.

High staff turnover in the childcare workforce has been prevalent for a number of years in England (Roberts 2011; Lloyd and Penn 2014; Elwick et al. 2018), in particular because of the rising higher qualification requirements to enter this profession that are nevertheless paired to persistently low salaries in the sector (Simon et al. 2015, 3; McDonald, Thorpe, and Irvine 2018). Parallel to the impact that austerity has had on state-maintained settings, the little value that carework and early years education holds, both at a societal level but also within institutions, were exemplified by these changes that the workforce at Ladybird faced. During fieldwork, I was reluctant to find out about some of the office politics that also seemed to play a part in most departures. Much of what I knew I gathered from coded remarks the staff made to each other about their issues with the school management, and whispered break room gossip, all of which was not particularly well hidden from me. Yet, it was nonetheless talk that was not intended for me to partake in, and neither did I feel comfortable doing so. During Joyce's leaving drinks in November, some specifics about the situation surfaced, including that a few of the nursery teachers did not feel like their work was being properly recognised and valued by their managers. This, they claimed, was partly due to the overemphasis on preparing children for primary education, which required them to record and assess children's progress in certain domains (mainly literacy and numeracy). The administrative labour that was required of them seemed to be taking over the other aspects of their jobs that they found more fulfilling. With the departure of these members of staff – Joyce, Robert, some of the lunchtime assistants, Emily, Brenda – the continuity and maintenance of caring relations within the Ladybird community seemed suddenly precarious.

What next for food policy and practice in early childhood education and care?

In this book, I have analysed the interaction of public health, education, and family intervention policies in early years settings in England, by exploring how feeding and eating practices unfolded within Ladybird Nursery and Children's Centre. In Chapter 1, I examined how the 'problems' of childhood obesity and high sugar intake have been framed in official discourse, taking into account perspectives from public health, early childhood education and care policy (ECEC), and the third (or charity) sector. Using Bacchi and Goodwin's 'What's the Problem Represented to be?' (WPR) approach (2016) I asked: what are the factors that are assumed to make the 'problems' persist? What is the historical context that underlies these assumptions? What is ignored in official framings of the 'problems'? What is the impact that official discourses had in people's daily lives? And, how do these representations of the 'problems' continue to hold authority in the public domain? Addressing these questions by analysing my ethnographic findings alongside secondary sources, I focused on the notions of responsibility and individual accountability that lie at the centre of these discourses. Subsequent chapters explored, inter alia, how these official framings of the 'problems' shaped feeding and eating practices at Ladybird and among families. In Chapter 2, responsibility and choice were also assessed in relation to the role that the food industry plays in determining people's diets, questioning the degree to which adults can limit children's consumption of certain foods.

Chapter 3 provided an account of the daily mealtime routines at Ladybird from the point of view of staff members. Exploring what the aims of feeding children in the early years were at the nursery, I examined the goals that most of the staff pursued during mealtimes at Ladybird, such as teaching children about 'healthy' eating and table manners. Parallel to this, I also explored the practical dimension of feeding children in an institutional setting, and the tensions that emerged between the logistical aspects of mealtimes and staff's personal ethics of care. Chapter 4 also focused on mealtime routines, this time from the perspective of the children. I showed that children created self- and peer-group identities through food and eating practices, predominantly through an exploration of their play behaviour, humour, and role reversal. I argued that children represented (and performed) food and mealtimes as channels through which to express care, enact authority, and communicate their knowledge about food and social relationships.

Chapter 5 moved on to an analysis of Ladybird as a provider of 'extended' (welfare) services to 'target parents,' by looking at the interactions that took place through three different interventions in the borough where I conducted fieldwork. By exploring the contradictions that emerged during these interventions, I challenged the official assumption that lack of knowledge and/or skills is one of the main barriers that low-income parents face when providing food to their children, arguing that material constraints should be instead properly accounted for in policy. Finally, Chapter 6 explored the theme of responsibility on a micro-level by analysing three mothers' accounts of self-scrutiny, and of trying to maintain control of their children's eating. I again showed the contrast between the universalism of official discourses about children's food (examined in Chapter 1) and the particularism that feeding children, and caring through food, requires. Simultaneously, I also explored the co-production of knowledge(s) and practices that adults and children are continuously engaged in. In discussing the norms that children brought with them from the school context into the home (and vice versa), and showing how these shaped adults' practices, I challenged the commonly held assumption that children's eating is unidirectionally influenced by adults.

Throughout the book, I have argued that the universalism of policy and bureaucracy – manifested in regulations, recommendations, the pursuit of measurable 'goals,' and audits – sits uncomfortably alongside the particularism of feeding children, at school and within the home environment. I have shown that adults, and 'policy communities' particularly, tend to pay most attention to *what* children eat, whilst to children it is *how* food is eaten that matters more. The limitations of nutrition-driven, individualistic approaches to food and eating were evidenced by examining the material constraints that both institutions and parents face when feeding children. Simultaneously, I have shown that the biomedical framing of food in nutritionial terms often draws attention away from its inherent social value, and its role in fostering and maintaining relationships of care.

My work is in conversation with that of other scholars who assess the unintended consequences of childcare and family policies that emerged particularly in the late 1990s (e.g. Clarke 2006; Camps and Long 2012; Sayer 2017) and under David Cameron's Conservative administration between 2010 and 2016 (e.g. Elliott and Hore 2016; Gillies, Edwards, and Horsley 2016, 2017). By providing an analysis that simultaneously assesses public health, ECEC, food, and family intervention policies, I have shown how assumptions travel between policy domains, and what the consequences of this are. Examining intergenerational relations on the ground level also reveals the strong role that generational power still plays in policy-related matters, as other scholars have shown (e.g. Tisdall 2016). This raises questions not only on how children can be included in policy (beyond tokenism), but also on what children's well-being might mean outside of an 'utilitarian' understanding of the concept (Tisdall 2015, 816).

In conducting this analysis of policy discourses and practices, I explored how the Mixed Economy of Welfare (MEW) (Powell 2014) functions on the ground within a domain that is under-researched in anthropology (the early years). Whilst on the one hand I problematised the implications of over-regulating, which emerge alongside audit culture, I also explored the consequences that come with the retreat of government from the public sector. The devolution of welfare services from the state to various non-governmental actors creates fragmentation in welfare provision, and gives space to knowledge(s) and practices that remain unaccountable to the communities that different organisations engage with. By extension, questioning who are the authoritative voices and the 'experts' in the children's food 'policy community' links to broader debates about what 'good food' is (e.g. Graf et al. 2019). Food, by extension, becomes a lens through which inequalities along class, ethnicity, gender, and, indeed, generational divisions can be examined closely. As Caplan argues, studying "food as a marker of difference" (1997, 9) contributes to an anthropological understanding not only of how people's eating practices are shaped and negotiated, but also acquire a moral dimension.

The accounts and viewpoints that emerged from my ethnography make it evident that feeding and caring are contingent on myriad circumstances that cannot be captured within the universalism of policy and bureaucracy. As Mol contends:

> Within the logic of care, trying to improve public health by persuading individuals to 'choose a healthy lifestyle' is not such a good idea. For a start, public health campaigns are too general, they make no differentiations. They

do not distinguish between specific people and their specific situations, but address us as if we were all equal [...] While addressing us as if we were equal, they do not provide care. Good care depends on specification.

(2008, 67)

Analysing food practices through the lens of care concretises the particularism and continuity that feeding and eating together require. Official and mainstream understandings of food practices are challenged, because these are always specific and dependent on context.

In thinking of care as an ongoing process (Mol 2008, 18), the continuous cycle of 'becoming' that we are all engaged in (and which depends on receiving care, through various channels) is also emphasised. Acknowledging this contribution emerging from the work of feminist scholars (e.g. Abel and Nelson 1990; Tronto 1993, 2013) problematises the still commonly held vision in policy and mainstream discourse that only children are 'becomings.' In fact, as numerous childhood scholars have previously made clear (see, e.g. Qvortrup 2005; Mayall 2006; Alanen 2011), children and adults alike are simultaneously 'beings' and 'becomings' (Uprichard 2008) – 'becoming' is a life-long process. Recognising this continuity is also to recognise that we all are vulnerable and need care. The challenge becomes to integrate this vision, and an understanding of the value of care (and the importance of maintaining stability in caring relations) to policymaking.

Over 20 years ago, Moss and Petrie suggested what some might consider a utopian solution that nonetheless was still cognizant of the realities of the UK sociopolitical climate, arguing that a small victory in moving towards better ECEC would be to rescind audit culture and the emphasis on 'measurable outcomes' in the sector (2000, 51). Drawing from the philosophies of the Reggio Emilia approach,[1] they argue that children's spaces, in contrast to the marketised notion of children's services, provide children with an opportunity to enter and engage with civic life (ibid., 115). Children are viewed as active agents whose contributions to the social worlds they engage in are properly recognised (ibid., 111). In this model, children's spaces are not simply places where 'efficient' citizens of the future are shaped, but where children's experiences in the present are valued, and creativity and critical thinking are encouraged. The notion that both children and adults are simultaneously 'beings' and 'becomings' lends itself well to this conceptualisation of children's spaces, for they are imagined as sites "for the *creation of common values* (for example, reciprocity), *rights...* and *culture*" (ibid., 115, original emphasis).

Whilst I do not intend to suggest that the Reggio Emilia approach could be easily imported and implemented in the English context, these considerations nonetheless could open up a range of possibilities for communities at large, of which children are a part but within which adults can also thrive. What if Sure Start Children's Centres (originally envisioned to support 'troubled families') existed, but not to 'improve' parenting practices, for example?

The same can be asked about food policy: what if the social value of food, rather than its categorisation as 'good' or 'bad,' were to be properly acknowledged in official discourse? As I showed in my ethnography, lack of knowledge and skills is not the main challenge that parents face when feeding their children, but material constraints are. These are not only financial, but time has also become a scarcer resource for parents in dual earning households, which have increasingly become the norm in Britain as in other nations (O'Connell and Brannen 2016). Enough evidence exists to suggest that nutrition-driven, market-based interventions can be lacking and contradictory (e.g. Cummins 2005; Caraher and Dowler 2007; Betty 2013; Evans 2017; Wake 2018), as I showed in Chapters 1 and 2 particularly. For example, in 2019 the 'Health, Exercise, Nutrition for the Really Young (HENRY) Approach' (Roberts 2015) received attention in the media exactly for this reason. At first hailed as an important solution to childhood obesity in Leeds, one of England's most impoverished areas (Boseley 2019), questions about the efficacy of targeting specific health matters without addressing the issue of socio-economic inequality at large (and its impact on the well-being of the population) later emerged (Vize 2019). Equally, the contradictions of promoting certain food standards and guide-lines within early years settings, whilst public funding for this sector is steadily being reduced (McDonald, Thorpe, and Irvine 2018; Early Years Alliance 2019), were also highlighted and addressed in this book.

A number of scholars have already suggested that a way to challenge these policy limitations is to champion a rights-based approach to address food insecurity (e.g. Dowler and O'Connor 2012). In these proposals, having access to sufficient and adequate food is framed as a matter of human dignity but also social inclusion – being able to share food with others is fundamental to human well-being. Rights-based approaches thus seek to hold states accountable when the material conditions for all households and institutions to access adequate and sufficient food are not in place, for example (ibid., 48). By a similar token, O'Connell, Knight, and Brannen have suggested that government policy that purports to address household food insecurity should "ensure that wages and welfare benefits, in combination, are adequate for a socially acceptable standard of living and eating" (2019, 128).

However, returning to the particular practices that emerge on a micro-level in people's daily lives, it is my hope that I have built a compelling case to argue that when closer attention is paid to what people deem meaningful about food and eating, the social value of food is elevated. Throughout this book, I have shown that if children are given the space – in the way that Moss and Petrie talk about children's spaces (2000) – children's self- and peer-group identities can flourish, which plays a fundamental role in maintaining their sense of well-being. Recognising that chil-dren and adults are simultaneously 'beings' and 'becomings' can help challenge the instrumental and pre-established boundaries that interactions and practices often acquire within an advanced liberal model.

Food is key to children's social participation – *what* they eat is just as important as *how* they eat. In line with a vision of children as agents, who learn by engaging freely with the multiple social worlds they inhabit, Andersen et al. propose a vision of 'food pedagogy' in which importance is given to "the voice of the child and 'learning by doing'" (Andersen, Baarts, and Holm 2017, 613). Through this approach, children can learn the political and ethical dimension of food, not just about health and nutrition, in a way that is linked to the rest of their daily activities.

Mealtimes can become the domains in which responsibility as reciprocity (Trnka and Trundle 2014) can be enacted. As I have demonstrated in this book, recognising children's agency and independence during mealtimes can allow for a number of situations to be resolved by them, as well as for interactions to be shaped and handled by children on their own terms. However, staff and parents are constrained by the material and discursive conditions that shape the competing agendas and priorities that different actors have when feeding children. Studying children's eating practices highlights the circularity and continuity on which caring relations rely, and the need for care and food to be better valued and acknowledged in future policy frameworks.

Note

1 "The Reggio Emilia approach to early childhood education…is based on the philosophies and practices of the infant-toddler centres of Reggio Emilia, Italy […] The school is viewed as a democratic place where the voices of all participants are valued and shaped by the experiences. Parents are active participants in the school and contribute valuable ideas, skills, and resources. The 'image of the child' is the belief that all children are capable, competent, powerful learners who bring to the school valuable theories and hypotheses of their own that are worthy of investigation. Learning is not linear and therefore not predictable. Teachers are keen observers of children and great importance is placed upon the adult being an active listener" (Shelley and Flessner 2013, 645–46).

References

Abel, Emily K., and Margaret K. Nelson. 1990. 'Circles of Care: An Introductory Essay'. In *Circles of Care: Work and Identity in Women's Life*, edited by Emily K. Abel and Margaret K. Nelson, 4–34. New York: State University of New York Press.

Andersen, Sidse Schoubye, Charlotte Baarts, and Lotte Holm. 2017. 'Contrasting Approaches to Food Education and School Meals'. *Food, Culture & Society* 20 (4): 609–29. https://doi.org/10.1080/15528014.2017.1357948.

Betty, A. L. 2013. 'Using Financial Incentives to Increase Fruit and Vegetable Consumption in the UK: Increasing Fruit and Vegetable Consumption'. *Nutrition Bulletin* 38 (4): 414–20. https://doi.org/10.1111/nbu.12062.

Boseley, Sarah. 2019. 'Leeds Becomes First UK City to Lower Its Childhood Obesity Rate'. *The Guardian*, 1 May 2019, sec. World news. http://www.theguardian.com/world/2019/may/01/leeds-becomes-first-uk-city-to-lower-its-childhood-obesity-rate.

Camps, Laura, and Tony Long. 2012. 'Origins, Purpose and Future of Sure Start Children's Centres'. *Nursing Children and Young People* 24 (1): 26–30.

Caplan, Pat. 1997. 'Approaches to the Study of Food, Health and Identity.' In *Food, Health, and Identity,* edited by Pat Caplan, 1–31. London: Routledge.

Caraher, Martin, and Elizabeth Dowler. 2007. 'Food Projects in London: Lessons for Policy and Practice—A Hidden Sector and the Need for "More Unhealthy Puddings… Sometimes"'. *Health Education Journal* 66 (2): 188–205.

Clarke, Karen. 2006. 'Childhood, Parenting and Early Intervention: A Critical Examination of the Sure Start National Programme'. *Critical Social Policy* 26 (4): 699–721. https://doi.org/10.1177/0261018306068470.

Cummins, S. 2005. 'Large Scale Food Retailing as an Intervention for Diet and Health: Quasi-Experimental Evaluation of a Natural Experiment'. *Journal of Epidemiology & Community Health* 59 (12): 1035–40. https://doi.org/10.1136/jech.2004.029843.

Dowler, Elizabeth A., and Deirdre O'Connor. 2012. 'Rights-Based Approaches to Addressing Food Poverty and Food Insecurity in Ireland and UK'. *Social Science & Medicine* 74 (1): 44–51. https://doi.org/10.1016/j.socscimed.2011.08.036.

Early Years Alliance. 2019. 'Early Years Funding Crisis "Hits Poorest Children"'. *Early Years Alliance - News* (blog). 11 June 2019. https://www.eyalliance.org.uk/news/2019/06/early-years-funding-crisis-hits-poorest-children.

Elliott, Victoria, and Beth Hore. 2016. '"Right Nutrition, Right Values": The Construction of Food, Youth and Morality in the UK Government 2010–2014'. *Cambridge Journal of Education* 46 (2): 177–93. https://doi.org/10.1080/0305764X.2016.1158785.

Elwick, Alex, Jayne Osgood, Leena Robertson, Mona Sakr, and Dilys Wilson. 2018. 'In Pursuit of Quality: Early Childhood Qualifications and Training Policy'. *Journal of Education Policy* 33 (4): 510–25. https://doi.org/10.1080/02680939.2017.1416426.

Evans, Charlotte Elizabeth Louise. 2017. 'Sugars and Health: A Review of Current Evidence and Future Policy'. *Proceedings of the Nutrition Society* 76 (03): 400–7. https://doi.org/10.1017/S0029665116002846.

Gillies, Val, Rosalind Edwards, and Nicola Horsley. 2016. 'Brave New Brains: Sociology, Family and the Politics of Knowledge'. *The Sociological Review* 64 (2): 219–37. https://doi.org/10.1111/1467-954X.12374.

———. 2017. *Challenging the Politcs of Early Intervention: Who's 'Saving' Children and Why*. Bristol: Policy Press.

Graf, Katharina, Anna Cohen, Brandi Simpson Miller, and Francesca Vaghi. 2019. 'Re-Examining the Contested Good: Proceedings from a Postgraduate Workshop on Good Food'. *Gastronomica: The Journal of Critical Food Studies* 19 (1): 91–93. https://doi.org/10.1525/gfc.2019.19.1.91.

Lloyd, Eva, and Helen Penn. 2014. 'Childcare Markets in an Age of Austerity'. *European Early Childhood Education Research Journal* 22 (3): 386–96. https://doi.org/10.1080/1350293X.2014.912901.

Mayall, Berry. 2006. 'Values and Assumptions Underpinning Policy for Children and Young People in England.' *Children's Geographies* 4 (1): 9–17. doi: 10.1080/14733280600576923

McDonald, Paula, Karen Thorpe, and Susan Irvine. 2018. 'Low Pay but Still We Stay: Retention in Early Childhood Education and Care'. *Journal of Industrial Relations* 60 (5): 647–68. https://doi.org/10.1177/0022185618800351.

Mol, Annemarie. 2008. *The Logic of Care: Health and the Problem of Patient Choice*. London: Routledge.

Moss, Peter, and Pat Petrie. 2000. *From Children's Services to Children's Spaces*. London: Routledge/Falmer.

O'Connell, Rebecca, and Julia Brannen. 2016. *Food, Families and Work*. London: Bloomsbury.

O'Connell, Rebecca, Abigail Knight, and Julia Brannen. 2016. *Living Hand to Mouth: Children and Food in Low-income Families*. London: Child Poverty Action Group.

Powell, Martin. 2014. *Understanding the Mixed Economy of Welfare*. Bristol: The Policy Press.

Qvortrup, Jens. 2005. 'Studies in Modern Childhood: Society, Agency, Culture'. In *Studies in Modern Childhood: Society, Agency, Culture,* edited by Jens Qvortrup, 1–20. Basinstoke: Palgrave Macmillan.

Roberts, Jonathan. 2011. 'Trust and Early Years Childcare: Parents' Relationships with Private, State and Third Sector Providers in England'. *Journal of Social Policy* 40 (4): 695–715. https://doi.org/10.1017/S0047279411000225.

Roberts, Kim. 2015. 'Growing Up Not out: The HENRY Approach to Preventing Childhood Obesity'. *British Journal of Obesity* 1 (3): 87–92.

Sayer, Andrew. 2017. 'Responding to the Troubled Families Programme: Framing the Injuries of Inequality'. *Social Policy and Society* 16 (01): 155–64. https://doi.org/10.1017/S1474746416000373.

Shelley, Ena, and Ryan Flessner. 2013. 'Reggio Emilia Approach'. In *Sociology of Education: An A-to-Z Guide*, edited by James Ainsworth 644–646. Thousand Oaks: SAGE Publications.

Simon, Antonia, Charlie Owen, Katie Hollingworth, and Jill Rutter. 2015. *Provision and Use of Preschool Childcare in Britain: Summary of Research Findings*. London: UCL Institute of Education.

Tisdall, E. Kay M. 2015. 'Children's Rights and Children's Wellbeing: Equivalent Policy Concepts?' *Journal of Social Policy* 44 (4): 807–23. doi:10.1017/S0047279415000306.

———. 2016.'Subjects with agency? Children's participation in family law proceedings.' *Journal of Social Welfare and Family Law* 38 (4): 362–79. doi: 10.1080/09649069.2016.1239345

Trnka, Susanna and Catherine Trundle. 2014. 'Competing Responsibilities: Moving Beyond Neoliberal Responsibilisation.' *Anthropological Forum* 24 (2): 136–53. doi: 10.1080/00664677.2013.879051

Tronto, Joan C. 1993. *Moral Boundaries: A Political Argument for an Ethic of Care*. New York: Routlegde.

———. 2013. 'Introduction: When Care Is No Longer 'at Home''. In *Caring Democracy. Markets, Equality, and Justice.* New York: New York University Press.

Uprichard, Emma. 2008. 'Children as "Being and Becomings": Children, Childhood and Temporality'. *Children & Society* 22 (4): 303–13. https://doi.org/10.1111/j.1099-0860.2007.00110.x.

Vize, Richard. 2019. 'Telling People to Eat Fewer Burgers Won't Solve Shocking Health Inequality'. *The Guardian*, 19 June 2019, sec. Society. https://www.theguardian.com/society/2019/jun/19/health-inequality-life-expectancy.

Wake, Melissa. 2018. 'The Failure of Anti-Obesity Programmes in Schools'. *BMJ* 360 (February): 1–2. https://doi.org/10.1136/bmj.k507.

Index

For Product Safety Concerns and Information please contact our EU
representative GPSR@taylorandfrancis.com
Taylor & Francis Verlag GmbH, Kaufingerstraße 24, 80331 München, Germany

www.ingramcontent.com/pod-product-compliance
Lightning Source LLC
Chambersburg PA
CBHW060306220326
41598CB00027B/4252

9 781032 286105